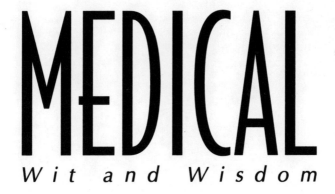

MEDICAL
Wit and Wisdom

Other books in this series:

"But I Wouldn't Want to Live There!"
by Michael Cader

The Little Library of Women's Wit and Wisdom

The Quotable Cat
by C.E. Crimmins

The Quotable Woman

Speaking of Baseball
by David Plaut

MEDICAL
Wit and Wisdom

The Best Medical Quotations

from Hippocrates to Groucho Marx

Compiled by Jess M. Brallier

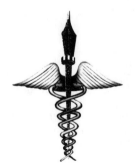

Running Press - Philadelphia, Pennsylvania

Canadian representatives: General Publishing Co., Ltd.,
30 Lesmill Road, Don Mills, Ontario M3B 2T6.

International representatives: Worldwide Media Services, Inc., 30
Montgomery Street, Jersey City, New Jersey 07302.

9 8 7 6 5 4 3 2 1
Digit on the right indicates the number of this printing.

Library of Congress Cataloging-in-Publication
Number 93-83465

ISBN 1-56138-289-2

Edited by Steven Zorn
Cover design by Toby Schmidt
Interior design by Stephanie Longo
Cover illustrations by Seth Jaben
Typography: Optima, with Bodega Sans, by Richard Conklin

This book may be ordered by mail from the publisher.
Please add $2.50 for postage and handling.
But try your bookstore first!
Running Press Book Publishers

DEDICATION

To my Mother, a dedicated nurse;
my Father, a caring dentist;
both, loving parents.

with special appreciation to Leigh Stoecker,
Curtis Vouwie, Alan Kellock, and as always, Sally

CONTENTS

Introduction

A good quote cuts right to the point, just like a skilled surgeon.

It is not at all surprising that so much of the world's most inspiring wisdom and enduring wit is rooted in medicine. Medicine addresses the extremes of the human condition—pain and comfort, loss and acceptance, tragedy and recovery, birth and death. Unlike the mechanic, bricklayer, or accountant, the medical practitioner has made it his or her life work to interact intimately with people who are at their most vulnerable. No wonder many observe life with such extraordinary clarity.

But the view from behind the surgeon's mask is decidedly different than the view from the operating table. No compilation of medical quotations would be complete without hearing from patients and other observers of the medical community.

Although medicine has changed over the years, the relationship between doctors and patients really hasn't. So the quotes in this book, whether they're about obstetrics, dermatology, or dentistry, and whether they originated in ancient Greece or in Montana last week, are equally apt. For more than 2,000 years, throughout six continents, a tenuous love-hate theme has permeated the healer-patient relationship.

Whichever side you're on, you're in good company. Erma Bombeck, Oliver Wendell Holmes, Benjamin Spock, Voltaire, Albert Schweitzer, Alfred Hitchcock, Mother Teresa, and others freely offer you their medical advice and opinions.

The message to all this is clearly, if you wish to be resented, pursue the medical profession. If, on the other hand, you hope to be admired and respected, certainly pursue the medical profession.

THE EXPERTS

The actress Billie Burke was dining in a restaurant where, at the next table, a man was obviously suffering from a bad cold.

"I can see you're very uncomfortable," she volunteered. "So I'll tell you what to do for it: drink lots of orange juice and take lots of aspirin. When you get to bed, cover yourself with as many blankets as you can find. Sweat the cold out. Believe me, I know what I'm talking about. I am Billie Burke of Hollywood."

The man smiled and introduced himself in return: "Thank you. I am Dr. Mayo of the Mayo Clinic."

The Human Condition

Birth, and copulation, and death.
That's all the facts when you come to brass tacks.

T.S. Eliot

Drinking when we are not thirsty and making love all year round, madam; that is all there is to distinguish us from other animals.

Pierre-Augustin Caron de Beaumarchais

Man appears to be the missing link between anthropoid apes and human beings.

Konrad Lorenz

We know the human brain is a device to keep the ears from grating on one another.

Peter De Vries

One can survive everything nowadays, except death.

Oscar Wilde

It is better to wear out than to rust out.

Richard Cumberland

Be happy while y'er leevin,
For y'er a lang time deid.

Scottish motto

Worry is the most natural and spontaneous of all human functions. It is time to acknowledge this, perhaps even to learn to do it better.

Lewis Thomas

Laughter is a form of internal jogging. It moves your internal organs around. It enhances respiration. It is an igniter of great expectations.

Norman Cousins

X rays: Their moral is this—that a right way of looking at things will see through almost anything.

Samuel Butler

The fate of a nation has often depended upon the good or bad digestion of a prime minister.

Voltaire

The healthy stomach is nothing if not conservative. Few radicals have good digestions.

Samuel Butler

Don't tell your friends about your indigestion:
"How are you!" is a greeting, not a question.

Arthur Guiterman

The best medicine I know for rheumatism is to thank the Lord
it ain't the gout.

Josh Billings

One hour's sleep before midnight, is worth two after.

Proverb

The amount of sleep required by the average person is just five
minutes more.

Anonymous

A good gulp of hot whiskey at bedtime—it's not very scientific,
but it helps.

Alexander Fleming

Early to rise and early to bed makes a male healthy and wealthy and dead.

James Thurber

The brain is a wonderful organ. It starts working the moment you get up in the morning, and does not stop until you get into the office.

Robert Frost

The average, healthy, well-adjusted adult gets up at seven-thirty in the morning feeling just plain terrible.

Jean Kerr

But Jesus, when you don't have any money, the problem is food. When you have money, it's sex. When you have both, it's health, you worry about getting ruptured or something. If everything is simply jake then you're frightened of death.

J.P. Donleavy

Life is one long process of getting tired.

Samuel Butler

Your vision will become clear only when you can look into your own heart. Who looks outside, dreams; who looks inside, awakes.

Carl Jung

Whatever comes from the brain carries the hue of the place it came from, and whatever comes from the heart carries the heat and color of its birthplace.

Oliver Wendell Holmes, Sr.

Ask many of us who are disabled what we would like in life and you would be surprised how few would say, "Not to be disabled." We accept our limitations.

Itzhak Perlman

Why does man have compassion for the blind
and for the deaf an irritable bind?

David Seegal

You can do anything with children if you only play with them.

Otto von Bismarck

It is so hard that one cannot really have confidence in doctors
and yet cannot do without them.

Johann Wolfgang von Goethe

It's no longer a question of staying healthy. It's a question of
finding a sickness you like.

Jackie Mason

When I began practice . . . I was relatively safe in assuming that abdominal pain was appendicitis or green apples. Today it is also highly probable that the patient is suffering from the fact that his wife of forty years wants to leave him for the Peace Corps or Richard Burton.

Gunnar Gundersen

I am convinced digestion is the great secret of life.

Sydney Smith

Every authority on etiquette discusses how to put things into your stomach, but very few discuss how to get them back out in a hurry. Actually, there is no way to make vomiting courteous. You have to do the next best thing, which is to vomit in such a way that the story you tell about it later will be amusing.

P.J. O'Rourke

You could say people are living longer because of the decline in religion. Not many people believe in the hereafter, so they keep going.

Cyril Clarke

We make ourselves sick by worrying about our health.

Lewis Thomas

There is no cure for birth and death save to enjoy the interval.

George Santayana

Knowledge

The great glory of modern medicine is that it regards nothing as essential but the truth.

Burton J. Hendrick

True science teaches, above all, to doubt and to be ignorant.

Miguel de Unamuno

It is with medicine as with mathematics: we should occupy our minds only with what we continue to know; what we once knew is of little consequence.

Charles Augustin Sainte-Beuve

The sound of a flute will cure epilepsy, and a sciatic gout.

Theophrastus

X rays are a hoax.

Lord Kelvin

Anatomy is to physiology as geography to history; it describes the theatre of events.

Jean Fernel

If th' Christyan Scientists had some science an' th' doctors more Christianity, it wudden't make anny diff'rence which ye called in—if ye had a good nurse.

Finley Peter Dunne

A good nurse is of more importance than a physician.

Hannah Farnham Lee

The trained nurse has become one of the great blessings of humanity, taking a place beside the physician and the priest, and not inferior to either in her mission.

William Osler

It is better to be sick than care for the sick.

Turkish proverb

I believe there is too strong a tendency on the part of so-called laymen to defer to the medical profession in regard to the [social] problems of medical care.

Carl J. Gilbert

The medical profession is unconsciously irritated by lay knowledge.

John Steinbeck

Matters of the Heart

It is infinitely better to transplant a heart than to bury it to be devoured by worms.

Christiaan N. Barnard

We all felt the majesty of the body . . . . As we saw the artificial heart beat . . . the feeling was not aren't we great, but aren't we small.

William C. DeVries

If you can think of how much love there would be in hundreds of hearts, then that is how much love there is in a plastic heart and when you grow up you will understand how very much love that is.

Michael E. De Bakey, answering a child who had asked, "Does a plastic heart have love in it?"

I would have picked up the artificial heart and thrown it on the floor and walked out and said he's dead if the press had not been there.

William C. DeVries, on the frustration of implanting the first artificial heart

Would you please turn on the television? I'd like to see if I'm still alive and how I'm doing.

Murray Haydon, artificial heart recipient

I wish Bill had written down on the consent form at what point he would want to say, "Stop this, I've had enough."

Margaret Schroeder, on her husband, an artificial-heart recipient, after he suffered a series of strokes

I despair of teaching the ordinary parent how to handle the child . . . . I would prefer to turn child-raising over to specialists.

B.F. Skinner

The greatest triumph of surgery today . . . lies in finding ways for avoiding surgery.

Robert Tuttle Morris

It is the malady of our age that the young are so busy teaching us that they have no time left to learn.

Eric Hoffer

Fashions in therapy may have some justification; fashions in diagnosis have none.

Charles Judson Herric

It is obvious that we cannot instruct women as we do men in the science of medicine; we cannot carry them into the dissecting room.

Walter Channing

Nowadays the clinical history too often weighs more than the man.

Martin H. Fischer

I don't give advice. I can't tell anybody what to do. Instead I say this is what we know about this problem at this time. And here are the consequences of these actions.

Joyce Brothers

Though we name the things we know, we do not necessarily know them because we name them.

Homer W. Smith

There was no influenza in my young days. We called a cold a cold.

Arnold Bennett

A genuine kiss generates so much heat it destroys germs.

S.L. Katzof

I really learned it all from mothers.

Benjamin Spock

The brain has muscles for thinking as the legs have muscles for walking.

Julien Offroy de la Mettrie

When a woman has scholarly inclinations there is generally something wrong with her sexual nature.

Friedrich Nietzsche

Critics

I am dying with the help of too many physicians.

Alexander the Great

The medical establishment has become a major threat to health.

Ivan Illich

It is astonishing with how little reading a doctor can practice medicine, but it is not astonishing how badly he may do it.

William Osler

Who ever said that doctors are truthful or even intelligent? You're getting a lot if they know their profession.

Majorie Karmel

Most people think that medical care is good for you. The fact is that some medical care is good for you, a great deal is irrelevant and, unfortunately, some of it is harmful.

Lester Breslow

He's a devout believer in the department of witchcraft called medical science.

George Bernard Shaw

Some day when you have time, look into the business of prayer, amulets, baths, and poultices, and discover for yourself how much valuable therapy the medical profession has cast out of the window.

Martin H. Fischer

It is . . . sometimes easier to head an institute for the study of child guidance than it is to turn one brat into a decent human being.

Joseph Wood Krutch

There are men who would even be afraid to commit themselves to the doctrine that castor oil is a laxative.

Camille Flammarion

Homeopathy is insignificant as an art of healing, but of great value as criticism on the hygeia or medical practice of the time.

Ralph Waldo Emerson

It would not be at all a bad thing if the elite of the medical world would be a little less clever, and would adopt a more primitive method of thinking, and reason more as children do.

George Groddeck

We may lay it down as a maxim, that when a nation abounds in physicians it grows thin of people.

Joseph Addison

Physicians are many in title but very few in reality.

Hippocrates

I often say a great doctor kills more people than a great general.

Gottfried Wilhelm von Leibniz

Many more Englishmen die by the lancet at home, than by the sword abroad.

John Armstrong

Physicians acquire their knowledge from our dangers, making experiments at the cost of our lives. Only a physician can commit homicide with impunity.

Pliny the Elder

Whenever he saw three physicians together, he looked up to discover whether there was not a turkey buzzard in the neighborhood.

Thomas Jefferson

Keep away from physicians. It is all probing and guessing and pretending with them. They leave it to Nature to cure in her own time, but they take the credit. As well as very fat fees.

Anthony Burgess

If you think that you have caught a cold, call in a good doctor. Call in three good doctors and play bridge.

Robert Benchley

With the exception of lawyers, there is no profession which considers itself above the law so widely as the medical profession.

Samuel Hopkins Adams

A Medical Glossary from
The Devil's Dictionary

by Ambrose Bierce

Apothecary, *n.* The physician's accomplice, undertaker's benefactor, and grave worm's provider.

Body Snatcher, *n.* A robber of grave worms. One who supplies the young physicians with that with which the old physicians have supplied the undertaker.

Brain, *n.* An apparatus with which we think that we think.

Dentist, *n.* A prestidigitator who, putting metal into your mouth, pulls coins out of your pocket.

Diagnosis, n. A physician's forecast of disease by the patient's pulse and purse.

Diaphragm, *n.* A muscular partition separating disorders of the chest from disorders of the bowels.

Gout, *n.* A physician's name for the rheumatism of a rich patient.

Grave, *n.* A place in which the dead are laid to await the coming of the medical student.

Heart, *n.* An automatic, muscular blood-pump. Figuratively, this useful organ is said to be the seat of emotions and sentiments—a very pretty fancy which, however, is nothing but a survival of a once universal belief. It is now known that the sentiments and emotions reside in the stomach.

Medicine, *n.* A stone flung down the Bowery to kill a dog on Broadway.

Physician, *n.* One upon whom we set our hopes when ill and our dogs when well.

The doctors are always changing their opinions. They always have some new fad.

David Lloyd George

A doctor is a man who writes prescriptions till the patient either dies or is cured by nature.

John Taylor

Life in itself is short enough, but the physicians with their art, know to their amusement how to make it still shorter.

Roger Bacon

The trouble with doctors is not that they don't know enough, but that they don't see enough.

Dominic J. Corrigan

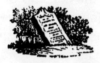

FROM CRADLE TO GRAVE

An elderly woman who had an ill-defined complaint and was a patient of Sir Walter Farquhar (1738-1819), believed that it would do her the world of good to take the waters at Bath for a few weeks.

Sir Walter encouraged her, and to allay her worries at the prospect of being separated from her usual physician, he promised to recommend her to a very clever doctor in Bath, a friend of his, and to write a letter for her to take with her, detailing her case.

The woman set out happily for Bath, but on the way began to think that although Sir Walter had been her physician for years, he had never told her precisely what was wrong with her. Her curiosity about the contents of the letter grew. At the first overnight stop she announced to her traveling companion that she was going to open it. Her companion protested about the breach of trust, but to no avail.

The letter was opened. It read: "Dear Davis, Keep the old lady three weeks and send her back again."

Sex and Reproduction

If a couple wishes to have a male child let the man take the womb and vulva of a hare and have it dried and pulverized; blend it with wine and let him drink it. Let the woman do the same with the testicles of the hare and let her be with her husband at the end of her menstrual period and she will conceive a male.

Trotula

One of the most obvious facts about grown-ups to a child is that they have forgotten what it is like to be a child.

Randall Jarrell

Parents learn a lot from their children about coping with life.

Muriel Spark

Adolescence is schizophrenia with a good prognosis.

Thomas L. Coleman

The mother-child relationship is paradoxical and, in a sense, tragic. It requires the most intense love on the mother's side, yet this very love must help the child grow away from the mother and to become fully independent.

Erich Fromm

Masturbation: the primary sexual activity of mankind. In the nineteenth century it was a disease; in the twentieth it's a cure.

Thomas Szasz

It is called in our schools "beastliness" and this is about the best name for it . . . should it become a habit it quickly destroys both health and spirits; he becomes feeble in body and mind, and often ends in a lunatic asylum.

Robert Baden-Powell

Masturbation produces seminal weakness, impotence, dysury, tabes dorsalis, pulmonary consumption, dyspepsia, dimness of sight, vertigo, epilepsy, hypochondriases, loss of memory, manalgia, fatuity, and death.

Benjamin Rush

Don't knock masturbation—it's sex with someone I love.

Woody Allen

We all worry about the population explosion, but we don't worry about it at the right time.

Arthur Hoppe

It serves me right for putting all my eggs in one bastard.

Dorothy Parker, on having an abortion

Copulation is dangerous immediately after a meal and during the two and three hours which the first digestion needs . . . .

Bernard S. Talmey

The greatest destroyer of peace is abortion because if a mother can kill her own child what is left for me to kill you and you to kill me? There is nothing between.

Mother Teresa

The mother of the year should be a sterilized woman with two adopted children.

Paul R. Ehrlich

I've noticed that everybody that is for abortion has already been born.

Ronald Reagan

It is now quite lawful for a Catholic woman to avoid pregnancy by a resort to mathematics, though she is still forbidden to resort to physics and chemistry.

H.L. Mencken

We want far better reasons for having children than not knowing how to prevent them.

Dora Russell

If men could get pregnant, abortion would be a sacrament.

Florynce Kennedy

They're borrowing one tiny little egg and some space.

Donna Regan, on being a surrogate mother

We need to make a world in which fewer children are born, and in which we take better care of them.

George Wald

It is as natural to die as to be born; and to a little infant, perhaps, the one is as painful as the other.

Francis Bacon

My mother groan'd, my father wept,
Into the dangerous world I lept;
Helpless, naked, piping loud,
Like a fiend hid in a cloud.

William Blake

If men had to have babies they would only ever have one each.

Diana, Princess of Wales

If nature had arranged that husbands and wives should have children alternatively, there would never be more than *three* in a family.

Laurence Housman

No man should marry until he has studied anatomy and dissected at least one woman.

Honoré de Balzac

It is not ultimately a matter of High Tech versus natural childbirth. The doctor does not necessarily always know best. A woman having a baby is doing what she was designed for and that equips her with a kind of knowing. Surely humility and respect on both sides is what is needed.

Mary Ellis

At the moment of childbirth, every woman has the same aura of isolation, as though she were abandoned, alone.

Boris Pasternak

There is nothing encourageth a woman sooner to be barren than hard travail in child bearing.

Pliny the Elder

A babe at the breast is as much pleasure as the bearing is pain.

Marion Zimmer Bradley

Parents are the last people on earth who ought to have children.

Samuel Butler

It's all any reasonable child can expect if the dad is present at the conception.

Joe Orton

The idea that birth can be both enjoyable and holy is immensely attractive.

Charles W. Thomas

The law of heredity is that all undesirable traits come from the other parent.

Anonymous

The history of man for the nine months preceding his birth would, probably, be far more interesting and contain events of greater moment than all the three score and ten years that follow it.

Samuel Taylor Coleridge

The management of fertility is one of the most important functions of adulthood.

Germaine Greer

Vasectomy means not ever having to say you're sorry.

Larry Adler

Being pregnant is a very boring six months. I am not particularly maternal.

Princess Anne

A society which practices death control must at the same time practice birth control.

John Rock

We have been God-like in our planned breeding of our domesticated plants and animals, but we have been rabbit-like in our unplanned breeding of ourselves.

Arnold Toynbee

Accidents will occur in the best-regulated families.

Charles Dickens

Marriages are not normally made to avoid having children.

Rudolf Virchow

What we desire our children to become, we must endeavour to be before them.

Andrew Combe

Maternity is a matter of fact—paternity is a matter of speculation.

H. Gideon Wells

Erection is chiefly caused by scuraum, eringoes, cresses, crymon, parsnips, artichokes, turnips, asparagus, candied ginger, acorns bruised to powder and drank in muscadel, scallion, sea shell fish, etc.

Aristotle

Like a slight attack of apoplexy.

Democritus, on orgasm

Take three pubic hairs and three from the left armpit. Burn them on a hot shovel. Pulverize and insert into a piece of bread. Dip bread in soup and feed to a lover.

Albertus Magnus, on a sure aphrodisiac

To win your beloved's affection: Take a piece of clothing into which you have freely perspired, and burn and powder it with some of your hair. Mix with your spit and blood and introduce it into the food and drink which your loved one will consume.

English folklore

The genitals themselves have not undergone the development of the rest of the human form in the direction of beauty.

Sigmund Freud

If a woman is normally developed mentally, and well-bred, her sexual desire is small. If this were not so, the whole world would become a brothel and marriage and a family impossible.

Joseph G. Richardson

It makes it possible for the sexual woman to act like a sexual man.

Marcus Crahan, on the birth control pill

What is a promiscuous person—it's usually someone who is getting more sex than you are.

Victor Lownes

Your sexuality is a dimension of your personality, and whenever you are sexually active, you are expressing yourself—the self that you are at that moment, the mood that you're in, the needs that you have.

Virginia Johnson

Sex is natural, but not if it's done right.

Woody Allen

Sex created the family.

Carl E. Fehrle

It is simply absurd that without modern science painless child-birth does not exist as a matter of course.

Isadora Duncan

I was caesarean born. You can't really tell, although whenever I leave a house, I go out through a window.

Steven Wright

Our biological drives are several million years older than our intelligence.

Arthur E. Morgan

If I had as many love affairs as you have given me credit for, I would now be speaking to you from a jar in the Harvard Medical School.

Frank Sinatra

Frigidity is the word used to describe impaired sexual feeling in women . . . and was probably coined by a man.

David M. Reuben

Male sexual response is far brisker and more automatic: it is triggered easily by things, like putting a quarter in a vending machine.

Alex Comfort

There's nothing wrong with your sex life that the right psycho-analyst can't exaggerate.

Laurence J. Peter

After the "change of life" with woman, sexual congress while permissible, should be infrequent, no less for her sake than that of the husband, whose advancing years should warn him of the medical maxim: "Each time that he delivers himself to this indulgence, he casts a shovelful of earth upon his coffin."

Nicholas Francis Cooke

I ask myself, in mercy, or in common sense, if we cannot alter the conviction to fit the body, should we not, in certain circumstances, alter the body to fit the conviction?

Harry Benjamin, to Jan Morris, who approached Benjamin for sex-change surgery

Some sexes change their sexes now
and make a mere man wonder how.

Alfred Kreymborg

Before the child ever gets to school it will have received crucial, almost irrevocable sex education and this will have been taught by the parents, who are not aware of what they are doing.

Mary S. Calderone

Sex is a natural function. You can't make it happen, but you can teach people to let it happen.

William H. Masters

You can't talk of the dangers of snake poisoning and not mention snakes.

C. Everett Koop, on the need to discuss sexual conduct as part of AIDS education

Sex is a pleasurable exercise in plumbing, but be careful or you'll get yeast in your drain tap.

Rita Mae Brown

Shed your clothes completely, and at the stroke of midnight
beneath a cloudless moon, walk three times around a house.
For each step you take, throw a handful of salt behind you. If
no one has seen you by the time you have finished, the person
you love will be mad for you.

Dutch aphrodisiac

Skullion had little use for contraceptives at the best of times.
Unnatural, he called them, and placed them in the lower
social category of things along with elastic-sided boots and
made-up bow ties. Not the sort of attire for a gentleman.

Tom Sharpe

The pleasure is momentary, the position ridiculous, and the
expense damnable.

Earl of Chesterfield

I'll wager you that in 10 years it will be fashionable again to be
a virgin.

Barbara Cartland

Poor honest sex, like dying, should be a private matter.

Laurence Durrell

If sex is such a natural phenomenon, how come there are so many books on how to?

Bette Midler

Sex is one of the nine reasons for reincarnation . . . the other eight are unimportant.

Henry Miller

The orgasm has replaced the Cross as the focus of longing and the image of fulfillment.

Malcolm Muggeridge

Love is two minutes fifty-two seconds of squishing noises. It shows your mind isn't clicking right.

Johnny Rotten

Love as a relation between men and women was ruined by the desire to make sure of the legitimacy of the children.

Bertrand Russell

Is it not strange that desire should so many years outlive performance?

William Shakespeare

Freud found sex an outcast in the outhouse and left it in the living room an honored guest.

W. Beran Wolfe

Women complain about sex more often than men. Their gripes fall into two major categories: 1) Not enough, 2) Too much.

Ann Landers

Certain times I like sex. Like after a cigarette.

Rodney Dangerfield

The sexual instinct is always active in woman whilst in man it is at rest from time to time.

Otto Weininger

One of the impressions from the East is that, in the West, we are obsessed with sex and romance [in our] plays, stories, songs, poetry, social customs.

Alan Gregg

Any scientist who has ever been in love knows that he may understand everything about sex hormones but the actual experience is something quite different.

Dame Kathleen Lonsdale

Whoever named it necking was a poor judge of anatomy.

Groucho Marx

Nature

Nature is that lovely lady to whom we owe polio, leprosy, smallpox, syphilis, tuberculosis, cancer.

Stanley N. Cohen

The art of medicine consists in amusing the patient while nature cures the disease.

Voltaire

If you believe in evolution, you can trace all of our lower back problems to the time when the first hominid stood erect. If you're a creationist, you can look at it this way: When Eve offered Adam the apple, he stood up to accept it.

Hugo A. Keim

Nature can refuse to speak but she cannot give a wrong answer.

Charles Brenton Huggins

One half of the children born die before their eighth year. This is nature's law; why try to contradict it?

Jean-Jacques Rousseau

You and your family must clearly understand that the great and ultimate healer is always nature itself and that the drug, the physician, and the patient can do no more than assist nature, by providing the very best conditions for your body to defend and heal itself.

Hans Krebs

Oh, the powers of nature. She knows what we need, and the doctors know nothing.

Benvenuto Cellini

The physician is only the servant of nature, not her master.
Therefore it behooves medicine to follow the will of nature.

Paracelsus

Employment is nature's physician, and is essential to human
happiness.

Galen

I've decided to skip "holistic." I don't know what it means, and
I don't want to know. That may seem extreme, but I followed
the same strategy toward "Gestalt" and the Twist, and lived to
tell the tale.

Calvin Trillin

The more man follows nature and is obedient to her laws, the
longer he will live; the further he deviates from these, the shorter will be his existence. Health is nature's reward for getting
into harmony with her laws.

Anita Hesselgesser

We have had for three weeks past a warm visit from the sun
(my almighty physician) and I find myself almost reestablished.

Thomas Jefferson

I have called this principle, by which each slight variation, if
useful, is preserved, by the term of Natural Selection.

Charles Darwin

Natural forces are the healers of disease.

Hippocrates

Nature heals, under the auspices of the medical profession.

Haven Emerson

The physician is Nature's assistant.

Galen

Man is Nature's sole mistake!

W.S. Gilbert

Health

Your health comes first—you can always hang yourself later.

Yiddish proverb

A rule of thumb in the matter of medical advice is to take everything any doctor says with a grain of aspirin.

Goodman Ace

When it comes to your health, I recommend frequent doses of that rare commodity among Americans—common sense.

Vincent Askey

I am in the habit of going to sea whenever I begin to grow hazy about the eyes, and to be over-conscious of my lungs.

Herman Melville

A man ought to handle his body like the sail of a ship, and neither lower and reduce it much when no cloud is in sight, nor be slack and careless in managing it when he comes to suspect something is wrong.

Plutarch

A healthy body is the guest-chamber of the soul, a sick, its prison.

Francis Bacon

Pain of mind is worse than pain of body.

Publilius Syrus

The greatest evil is physical pain.

St. Augustine

Your heaviest artillery will be your will to live. Keep that big gun going.

Norman Cousins

You want to go easy on the suicide stuff—first thing you know, you'll ruin your health.

Robert Benchley

Health is the first muse, and sleep is the condition to produce it.

Ralph Waldo Emerson

Sleep is that golden chain that ties health and our bodies together.

Thomas Dekker

The ancient inhabitants of this island were less troubled with coughs when they went naked, and slept in caves and woods, than men now in chambers and feather-beds.

Thomas Browne

The Prognosis

Oliver Wendell Holmes, Sr., the writer and physician, arrived at the house of a poor patient one morning to find the priest about to depart.

"Your patient is very ill," said the priest solemnly, "he is going to die."

Holmes nodded, "Yes, and he's going to hell."

The priest was horrified, "I have just given him extreme unction! You must not say such things!"

Holmes shrugged his shoulders, "Well, you expressed a medical opinion and I have just as much right to a theological opinion."

Fresh air impoverishes the doctor.

Danish proverb

Bathe twice a day to be really clean, once a day to be passably clean, once a week to avoid being a public menace.

Anthony Burgess

Three things give hardy strength: sleeping on hairy mattresses, breathing cold air, and eating dry food.

Welsh proverb

A man who fears suffering is already suffering from what he fears.

Michel de Montaigne

Study sickness while you are well.

Thomas Fuller

People who are always taking care of their health are like misers, who are hoarding a treasure which they have never spirit enough to enjoy.

Laurence Sterne

It is better to lose health like a spendthrift than to waste it like a miser, better to live and be done with it, than to die daily in the sick room.

Robert Louis Stevenson

The poorest man would not part with health for money, but the richest would gladly part with all their money for health.

Charles Caleb Cotton

The view that a peptic ulcer may be the hole in a man's stomach through which he crawls to escape from his wife has fairly wide acceptance.

J.A.D. Anderson

Health is the thing that makes you feel that now is the best time of the year.

Franklin P. Adams

The health of people is really the foundation upon which all their happiness and all their power as a State depend.

Benjamin Disraeli

If I had my way I'd make health catching instead of disease.

Robert G. Ingersoll

Thousands upon thousands of persons have studied disease. Almost no one has studied health.

Adelle Davis

'Tis healthy to be sick sometimes.

Henry David Thoreau

Health is not a condition of matter, but of Mind; nor can the material senses beat reliable testimony on the subject of health.

Mary Baker Eddy

There is no curing a sick man who believes himself in health.

Henri Amiel

Quit worrying about your health. It'll go away.

Robert Orben

Men who pass most comfortably through the world are those who possess good digestions and hard hearts.

Harriet Martineau

He who drinks a tumbler of London water has literally in his stomach more animated beings than there are men, women, and children on the face of the globe.

Sydney Smith

Of all cooperative enterprises public health is the most important and gives the greatest returns.

William J. Mayo

Public health is purchasable. Within natural limitations any
community can determine its own death rate.

Hermann M. Biggs

It is a lot harder to keep people well than it is to just get them
over a sickness.

DeForest Clinton Jarvis

Sleep, riches, and health, to be truly enjoyed, must be inter-
rupted.

Jean Paul Richter

Life is not living, but living in health.

Martial

Aging

My diseases are an asthma and a dropsy and, what is less curable, seventy-five.

Samuel Johnson

I don't deserve this award, but I have arthritis and I don't deserve that either.

Jack Benny

No skill or art is needed to grow old; the trick is to endure it.

Johann Wolfgang von Goethe

It is not by muscle, speed, or physical dexterity that great things are achieved, but by reflection, force of character, and judgement; in these qualities old age is usually not only not poorer, but is even richer.

Cicero

You will recognize, my boy, the first sign of old age: it is when you go out into the streets of London and realize for the first time how young the policemen look.

Seymour Hicks

As for me, except for an occasional heart attack, I feel as young as I ever did.

Robert Benchley

The misery of a child is interesting to a mother, the misery of a young man is interesting to a young woman, the misery of an old man is interesting to nobody.

Victor Hugo

A medical revolution has extended the life of our elder citizens without providing the dignity and security those later years deserve.

John F. Kennedy

Life is precious to the old person. He is not interested merely in thoughts of yesterday's good life and tomorrow's path to the grave. He does not want his later years to be a sentence of solitary confinement in society. Nor does he want them to be a death watch.

David Allman

The ageing man of the middle twentieth century lives, not in the public world of atomic physics and conflicting ideologies, of welfare states and supersonic speed, but in his strictly private universe of physical weakness and mental decay.

Aldous Huxley

Old age puts more wrinkles in our minds than on our faces.

Michel de Montaigne

Old age is an island surrounded by death.

Juan Montalvo

Man arrives as a novice at each age of his life.

Nicholas Chamfort

Youth is a blunder; manhood a struggle; old age a regret.

Benjamin Disraeli

At sixteen I was stupid, confused, insecure, and indecisive. At twenty-five I was wise, self-confident, prepossessing, and assertive. At forty-five I am stupid, confused, insecure, and indecisive. Who would have supposed that maturity is only a short break in adolescence?

Jules Feiffer

We do not necessarily improve with age: for better or worse we become more like ourselves.

Peter Hall

The four stages of man are infancy, childhood, adolescence, and obsolescence.

Art Linkletter

I am just turning 40 and taking my time about it.

Harold Lloyd, at 77

To me, old age is always 15 years older than I am.

Bernard Baruch

Do you think my mind is maturing late,
Or simply rotted early?

Ogden Nash, at 40

From birth to age 18, a girl needs good parents. From 18 to 35, she needs good looks. From 35 to 55, she needs a good personality. From 55 on, she needs good cash.

Sophie Tucker

Years ago we discovered the exact point at the dead centre of middle age. It occurs when you are too young to take up golf and are too old to rush up to the net.

Franklin P. Adams

Middle age is when your age starts to show around the middle.

Bob Hope

In a man's middle years there is scarcely a part of the body he would hesitate to turn over to the proper authorities.

E.B. White

Aging seems to be the only available way to live a long time.

Deaniel-François-Esprit Auber

An old man looks permanent, as if he had been born an old man.

H.E. Bates

I smoke 10 to 15 cigars a day, at my age I have to hold on to something.

George Burns

When I was 40, my doctor advised me that a man in his forties shouldn't play tennis. I heeded his advice carefully and could hardly wait until I reached 50 to start again.

Hugo Black

Forty is the old age of youth; fifty is the youth of old age.

French proverb

The denunciation of the young is a necessary part of the hygiene of older people, and greatly assists the circulation of their blood.

Logan Pearsall Smith

A majority of young people seem to develop mental arteriosclerosis 40 years before they get the physical kind.

Aldous Huxley

Youth is a malady of which one becomes cured a little every day.

Benito Mussolini

Youth is a wonderful thing. What a crime to waste it on children.

George Bernard Shaw

A physician can sometimes parry the scythe of death, but has no power over the sand in the hourglass.

Hester Lynch Piozzi

Prescriptions for Longevity

Swim, dance a little, go to Paris every August and live within walking distance of two hospitals.

Horatio Luro, at 80

Stay busy, get plenty of exercise and don't drink too much.
Then again, don't drink too little.

Herman "Jackrabbit" Smith-Johannsen, at 103

There is no short-cut to longevity. To win it is the work of a lifetime, and the promotion of it is a branch of preventive medicine.

James Crichton-Browne

Time carries all things, even our wits, away.

Virgil

Body and mind, like man and wife, do not always agree to die together.

Charles C. Colton

Our lives are like a candle in the wind.

Carl Sandburg

First thing I do when I wake up in the morning is breathe on a mirror and hope it fogs.

Earl Wynn

Mental activity increases throughout adult life—*if* the mind is kept active, interested, and useful. It will decrease by inactivity, not by aging.

Hardin B. Jones

The body never lies.

Martha Graham

I have everything now I had 20 years ago—except now it's all lower.

Gypsy Rose Lee

Age will not be defied.

Francis Bacon

In the morning, we carry the world like Atlas; at noon, we stoop and bend beneath it; and at night, it crushes us flat to the ground.

Henry Ward Beecher

A man is as old as his arteries.

Thomas Sydenham

Live as long as you may, the first twenty years are the longest half of your life.

Robert Southey

Physically, a man is a man for a much longer time than a woman is a woman.

Honoré de Balzac

Tobacco, coffee, alcohol, hashish, prussic acid, strychnine, are weak dilutions: the surest poison is time.

Ralph Waldo Emerson

Middle age has been said to be the time of a man's life when, if he has two choices for an evening, he takes the one that gets him home earlier.

Alvan L. Barach

We have, inadvertently, trained our young doctors to consider it a virtue to prolong life for the sole purpose of prolonging it.

James Howard Means

As I grow older, I have less and less sympathy with the conscientious efforts merely to extend life in old age.

Warfield T. Longcope

I inhabit a weak, frail, decayed tenement; battered by the winds and broken in on by the storms, and, from all I can learn, the landlord does not intend to repair.

John Quincy Adams

I prefer old age to the alternative.

Maurice Chevalier

Smoking and Other Vices

Smoking is, as far as I am concerned, the entire point of being an adult.

Fran Lebowitz

It is in the interests of society to put the Pill into vending machines and to place cigarettes on prescription.

Malcolm Potts

An alcoholic has been lightly defined as a man who drinks more than his own doctor.

Alvan L. Barach

It was my Uncle George who discovered that alcohol was a food well in advance of modern medical thought.

P.G. Wodehouse

If your doctor warns that you have to watch your drinking, find a bar with a mirror.

John Mooney

The brewery is the best drugstore.

German proverb

If you drink, don't drive. Don't even putt.

Dean Martin

I never smoked a cigarette until I was nine.

H.L. Mencken

Smokers, male and female, inject and excuse idleness in their lives every time they light a cigarette.

Colette

The strongest possible piece of advice I would give to any young woman is: Don't screw around, and don't smoke.

Edwina Currie

But when I don't smoke I scarcely feel as if I'm living. I don't feel as if I'm living unless I'm killing myself.

Russell Hoban

A custom loathsome to the eye, hateful to the nose, harmful to the brain, dangerous to the lungs, and in the black, stinking fume thereof, nearest resembling the horrible Stygian smoke of the pit that is bottomless.

James I

Smoking . . . is a shocking thing, blowing smoke out of our mouths into other people's mouths, eyes and noses, and having the same thing done to us.

Samuel Johnson

Selling Smokes

Not a cough in a carton.

Old Gold

The throat-tested cigarette.

Philip Morris

Nose, throat, and accessory organs not adversely affected.

Chesterfield

More doctors smoke Camels than any other cigarette.

Camel

Smoking shortens your life by eight years. I love watching pro football on television. If I smoke, I'll miss 350 games.

Tony Curtis

I have every sympathy with the American who was so horrified by what he had read of the effects of smoking that he gave up reading.

Henry G. Strauss

When I was young, I kissed my first woman, and smoked my first cigarette on the same day. Believe me, never since have I wasted any more time on tobacco.

Arturo Toscanini

A woman is only a woman, but a good cigar is a smoke.

Rudyard Kipling

Tobacco drieth the brain, dimmeth the sight, vitiateth the smell, hurteth the stomach, destroyeth the concoction, disturbeth the humors and spirits, corrupteth the breath, induceth a trembling of the limbs, exiccateth the windpipe, lungs and liver, annoyeth the milt, scorcheth the heart, and causeth the blood to be adjusted.

Tobias Venner

Cigarette smoking is clearly identified as the chief preventable cause of death in our society.

C. Everett Koop

Woman died at Savannah, Georgia, age 123. She had smoked a pipe for 112 years, while cigarette smokers figure they are passing out daily at the ripe old age of thirty or forty. I think it's the fatigue from tapping 'em on the cigarette case that wears 'em down so early.

Will Rogers

In a smoker, probably the earliest known indication of disease is that he begins to give up tobacco.

Richard Clarke Cabot

A major error of the current drug classification system is that it treats alcohol and nicotine—two of the most harmful drugs—essentially as nondrugs.

Edward M. Brecher

Make it legal and the cigarette companies will come in and put filter tips on your pot and vitamins and menthol in your pot. No. I say keep it criminal.

Norman Mailer

There are people who strictly deprive themselves of each and every eatable, drinkable and smokable which has in any way acquired a shady reputation. They pay this price for health. And health is all they get for it.

Mark Twain

Every form of addiction is bad, no matter whether the narcotic
be alcohol or morphine or idealism.

Carl Jung

■

Exercise and Diet

How much happiness is gained, and how much misery
escaped, by frequent and violent agitation of the body.

Samuel Johnson

If God had intended man to engage in strenuous sports, He
would have given us better knees.

Robert Ray

All that running and exercise can do for you is make you healthy.

Denny McLain

I get my exercise acting as a pallbearer to my friends who exercised.

Chauncey Depew

Health food makes me sick.

Calvin Trillin

We sit at breakfast, we sit on the train on the way to work, we sit at work, we sit at lunch, we sit all afternoon . . . a hodge-podge of sagging livers, sinking gallbladders, drooping stomachs, compressed intestines and squashed pelvic organs.

John Button, Jr.

We can now prove that large numbers of Americans are dying from sitting on their behinds.

Bruce B. Dan

A man ought to have a doctor's prescription to be allowed to use a golf cart.

Paul Dudley White

We are under-exercised as a nation. We look instead of play. We ride instead of walk. Our existence deprives us of the minimum of physical activity essential for healthy living.

John F. Kennedy

People are the only animals who eat themselves to death.

The American Medical Association

We tolerate shapes in human beings that would horrify us if we saw them in a horse.

W.R. Inge

Attributing overweight to overeating is hardly more illuminating than ascribing alcohol to alcoholism.

Jean Mayer

Has it ever struck you that there's a thin man inside every fat man, just as they say there's a statue inside every block of stone?

George Orwell

Outside every fat man there is an even fatter man trying to close in.

Kingsley Amis

Health nuts are going to feel stupid someday, lying in a hospital dying of nothing.

Redd Foxx

If your eyes are set wide apart you should be a vegetarian, because you inherit the digestive characteristics of bovine or equine ancestry.

Linard Williams

Vegetarians have wicked, shifty eyes and laugh in a cold, calculating manner. They pinch little children, steal stamps, drink water, favor beards.

J.B. Morton

Persons living very entirely on vegetables are seldom of a plump and succulent habit.

William Cullen

Vegetarianism is harmless enough though it is apt to fill a man with wind and self-righteousness.

Robert Hutchison

I did not become a vegetarian for my health. I did it for the health of the chickens.

Isaac Bashevis Singer

Food is an important part of a balanced diet.

Fran Lebowitz

I told my doctor I get very tired when I go on a diet, so he gave me pep pills. Know what happened? I ate faster.

Joe E. Lewis

The Chinese do not draw any distinction between food and medicine.

Lin Yutang

Kitchen Physic is the best Physic.

Jonathan Swift

A food is not necessarily essential just because your child hates it.

Katherine Whitehorn

I believe every human has a finite number of heartbeats. I don't intend to waste any of mine running around doing exercises.

Neil Armstrong

Exercise is bunk. If you are healthy, you don't need it; if you are sick, you shouldn't take it.

Henry Ford

It's unnatural for people to run around city streets unless they are thieves or victims. It makes people nervous to see someone running. I know that when I see someone running on my street, my instincts tell me to let the dog out after him.

Mike Royko

A vigorous five-mile walk will do more good for an unhappy but otherwise healthy adult than all the medicine and psychology in the world.

Paul Dudley White

A high-fiber breakfast is very important. Always eat your cereal before it shrinks.

Mark Russell

Those who think they have not time for bodily exercise will sooner or later have to find time for illness.

Edward Stanley

Gluttony is an emotional escape, a sign something is eating us.

Peter De Vries

In eating, a third of the stomach should be filled with food, a third with drink, and the rest left empty.

The Talmud

Doctors are always working to preserve our health and cooks to destroy it, but the latter are more often successful.

Denis Diderot

A man of sixty has spent twenty years in bed and over three years eating.

Arnold Bennett

Wine is the most healthful and most hygienic of beverages.

Louis Pasteur

We drink one another's health and spoil our own.

Jerome K. Jerome

Drink a glass of wine after your soup, and you steal a ruble from the doctor.

Russian proverb

Death on the expense account is a characteristic feature of the affluent society.

René J. Dubos

A glutton digs his grave with his teeth.

French proverb

Not less than two hours a day should be devoted to exercise.

Thomas Jefferson

The longer I live the less confidence I have in drugs and the greater is my confidence in the regulation and administration of diet and regimen.

John Redman Coxe

Immature faddists are continuously proclaiming the value of exercise: four people out of five are more in need of rest than exercise.

Logan Clendening

He neither drank, smoked, nor rode a bicycle. Living frugally, saving his money, he died early, surrounded by greedy relatives. It was a great lesson to me.

John Barrymore

Teetotalers lack the sympathy and generosity of men that drink.

W.H. Davies

Two out of every three deaths are premature: they are related to loafer's heart, smoker's lung, and drinker's liver.

Thomas J. Bassler

Illness and Disease

Illness is the doctor to whom we pay most heed: to kindness, to knowledge we make promises only; pain we obey.

Marcel Proust

The most important thing in illness is never to lose heart.

Nikolai Lenin

Many illnesses are promoted from the third-rate to the first-rate by the anxious mind.

Eric Partridge

The sorrow which has no vent in tears may make other organs weep.

Henry Maudsley

Thinking is the most unhealthy thing in the world, and people die of it just as they die of any other disease.

Oscar Wilde

Illnesses must be regarded as a madness of the body, indeed as idées fixes.

Friedrich von Hardenberg

Body and soul cannot be separated for purposes of treatment, for they are one and indivisible. Sick minds must be healed as well as sick bodies.

C. Jeff Miller

A bodily disease, which we look upon as whole and entire within itself, may, after all, be but a symptom of some ailment in the spiritual part.

Nathaniel Hawthorne

All of us are mad. If it weren't for the fact that every one of us is slightly abnormal, there wouldn't be any point in giving each person a separate name.

Ugo Betti

If you are physically sick, you can elicit the interest of a battery of physicians; but if you are mentally sick, you are lucky if the janitor comes around.

Martin H. Fischer

The diseases of the mind are more destructive than those of the body.

Marcus Tullius Cicero

The proclivity of extraordinary violence is not just an ailment of the mind, as psychologists like to think. Nor is it only a malaise of the society, as sociologists believe. It is both of these things, but it is also a sickness of the body as distinct and definite as cancer or leprosy.

Vernon H. Mark

Don't wake him up. He's got insomnia. He's trying to sleep it off.

Chico Marx

We don't believe in rheumatism and true love until after the first attack.

Marie Von Ebner-Eschenbach

Love's a disease. But curable.

Rose Macaulay

Life is an incurable disease.

Abraham Cowley

I enjoy convalescence. It is the part that makes the illness worthwhile.

George Bernard Shaw

Physical ills are the taxes laid upon this wretched life; some are taxed higher, and some lower, but all pay something.

Philip Stanhope Chesterfield

How sickness enlarges the dimensions of a man's self to himself! He is his own exclusive object . . . . He has nothing to think of but how to get well.

Charles Lamb

When you get that close to the abyss, you can always jump tomorrow.

Ian Lustbader

The diseases of the present have little in common with the diseases of the past save that we die of them.

Duke of Richelieu

For epilepsy in adults I recommend spirit of human brain or a powder, to be compounded only in May, June, and July, from the livers of live green frogs.

Johann Hartmann

We all labor against our own cure, for death is the cure of all diseases.

Thomas Browne

The soul's maladies have their relapses like the body's. What we take for a cure is often just a momentary rally or a new form of the disease.

François Duc de la Rochefoucauld

To avoid sickness, eat less; to prolong life, worry less.

Chu Hui Weng

All that wheezes is not asthma.

Chevalier Jackson

Did you ever have the measles, and if so, how many?

Artemus Ward

Jaundice is the disease that your friends diagnose.

William Osler

He who scratches a scar is wounded twice.

Russian proverb

The trouble with heart disease is that the first symptom is often hard to deal with: sudden death.

Michael Phelps

We are sick because our cells are sick.

Christian de Duve

It's just like remodeling an office. The body tears out partitions, puts up dry walls and paints.

Robert P. Heaney, on how the body takes calcium from bones when there is a shortage in the blood

A cancer is not only a physical disease, it is a state of mind.

Michael M. Baden

Clearly, if disease is manmade, it can also be man-prevented. It should be the function of medicine to help people die young as late in life as possible.

Ernst Wudner

Serious illness doesn't bother me for long because I am too inhospitable a host.

Norman Cousins

Women agonize . . . over cancer; we take as personal threat the lump in every friend's breast.

Martha Weinman Lear

I am not going to fight against death but for life.

Norbert Segard

She was losing her mind in handfuls.

Marion Roach, on her mother, a victim of Alzheimer's disease

Disease makes men more physical, it leaves them nothing but body.

Thomas Mann

Children, in general, are overclothed and overfed. To these causes, I impute most of their diseases.

William Cadogan

When meditating over a disease, I never think of finding a remedy for it, but, instead, a means of preventing it.

Louis Pasteur

There are only two things a child will share willingly—communicable diseases and his mother's age.

Benjamin Spock

The deviation of man from the state in which he was originally placed by nature seems to have proved to him a prolific source of diseases.

Edward Jenner

Decay and disease are often beautiful, like the pearly tear of the shellfish and the hectic glow of consumption.

Henry David Thoreau

Despite a lifetime of service to the cause of sexual liberation I have never caught a venereal disease, which makes me feel rather like an arctic explorer who has never had frostbite.

Germaine Greer

Two minutes with Venus, two years with mercury.

J. Earle Moore

You're not sleeping with one person, you're sleeping with everyone they ever slept with.

Theresa Crenshaw, on AIDS

We're all going to go crazy, living this [AIDS] epidemic every minute, while the rest of the world goes on out there, all around us, as if nothing is happening, going on with their own lives and not knowing what it's like, what we're going through. We're living through war, but where they're living it's peacetime, and we're all in the same country.

Larry Kramer

Epidemics have often been more influential than statesmen and soldiers in shaping the course of political history, and diseases may also color the moods of civilizations.

René Dubos

Some people are so sensitive they feel snubbed if an epidemic overlooks them.

Frank Hubbard

All diseases of Christians are to be ascribed to demons.

St. Augustine

In the nineteenth century men lost their fear of God and acquired a fear of microbes.

Anonymous

The Diagnosis

Samuel Morse, inventor of the telegraph, was also an accomplished artist. He once painted a picture of a man in his death agony and showed it to a friend who happened to be a doctor.

"Well, what's your opinion?" Morse demanded, after his friend had studied the painting.

"Malaria," said the physician without hesitation.

They do certainly give very strange and new-fangled names to diseases.

Plato

Physicians think they do a lot for a patient when they give his disease a name.

Immanuel Kant

The fact that your patient gets well does not prove that your diagnosis was correct.

Samuel J. Meltzer

The doctor may also learn more about the illness from the way the patient tells the story than from the story itself.

James B. Herrick

For the most violent diseases the most violent remedies.

Michel de Montaigne

When a young physician he possessed twenty remedies for every disease, and at the close of his career he found twenty diseases for which he had not one remedy.

John Radcliffe

Pathologists have long known . . . that rheumatic fever "licks at the joints, but bites at the heart."

Ernest Charles Lasegue

Like an earthquake, true senility announces itself by trembling and stammering.

Santiage Ramon y Cajal

All the vast hygienic, social and moral problems of our restless, energetic labor-saving race are, in some degree, those of the future student of disease in America.

Weir Mitchell

Hypochondria

We are rapidly becoming a land of hypochondriacs, from the ulcer-and-martini executives in the big city to the patent medicine patrons in the sulfur-and-molasses belt.

Vincent Askey

It is the manner of hypochondriacs to change often their physician . . . for a physician who does not admit the reality of the disease cannot be supposed to take much pains to cure it.

William Cullen

The best cure for hypochondria is to forget about your body and get interested in somebody else's.

Goodman Ace

Hypochondriacs squander large sums of time in search of nostrums by which they vainly hope they may get more time to squander.

Charles C. Colton

Hungry Joe collected lists of fatal diseases and arranged them in alphabetical order so that he could put his finger without delay on any one he wanted to worry about.

Joseph Heller

I never read a patent medicine advertisement without being impelled to the conclusion that I am suffering from the particular disease therein dealt with in its most virulent form.

Jerome K. Jerome

Hypochondria: The imaginary complaints of indestructible old ladies.

E.B. White

■

Death

A doctor's reputation is made by the number of eminent men who die under his care.

George Bernard Shaw

Death . . . a friend that alone can bring the peace his treasures cannot purchase, and remove the pain his physicians cannot cure.

Charles C. Colton

My doctor gave me two weeks to live. I hope they're in August.

Ronnie Shakes

When a man lies dying, he does not die from the disease alone. He dies from his whole life.

Charles Péguy

Why, he that cuts off twenty years of life
Cuts off so many years of fearing death.

William Shakespeare

After all, what is death? Just nature's way of telling us to slow down.

Dick Sharples

Death must be distinguished from dying, with which it is often confused.

Sydney Smith

It hath been often said, that it is not death, but dying, which is terrible.

Henry Fielding

Death is a delightful hiding-place for weary men.

Herodotus

On his deathbed, British surgeon Joseph Henry Green behaved very coolly. "Congestion," he observed, and then took his own pulse. "Stopped," he said, and died.

Death is a punishment to some, to some a gift, and to many a favour.

Seneca

Death is not the greatest of ills, it is worse to want to die, and not to be able to.

Sophocles

Either this man is dead or my watch has stopped.

Groucho Marx

It is impossible that anything so natural, so necessary, and so universal as death, should ever have been designed by Providence as an evil to mankind.

Jonathan Swift

How beautiful the body is . . . . How terrible when torn. The little flame of life sinks lower and lower and, with a flicker, goes out. It goes out like a candle goes out. Quietly and gently. It makes its protest at extinction, then submits. It has its say, then is silent.

Norman Bethune

Watching a peaceful death of a human being reminds us of a falling star; one of a million lights in a vast sky that flares up for a brief moment only to disappear into the endless night forever.

Elisabeth Kübler-Ross

You do not die all at once. Some tissues live on for minutes, even hours, giving still their little cellular shrieks, molecular echoes of the agony of the whole corpus.

Richard Selzer

You die as you've lived. If you were paranoid in life, you'll probably be paranoid when you're dying.

James Cimino

The death of a child is the single most traumatic event in medicine. To lose a child is to lose a piece of yourself.

Burton Grebin

Any man's death diminishes me, because I am involved in
      Mankinde;
And therefore never send to know for whom the bell tolls;
It tolls for thee.

John Donne

Famous Last Words

Either they go, or I do.

Oscar Wilde, of his new bedroom curtains

If this is dying, I don't think much of it.

Lytton Strachey

Moose! . . . Indians!

Henry David Thoreau

I'm dying, but otherwise I'm in very good health.

Edith Sitwell

Die, my dear doctor! That's the last thing I shall do!

Lord Palmerston

This is the last of earth! I am content!

John Quincy Adams

So little done, so much to do.

Cecil Rhodes

Is this dying? Is this all? Is this all that I feared, when I prayed against a hard death? Oh, I can bear this! I can bear it! I can bear it!

Cotton Mather

Death is the poor man's best physician.

Irish proverb

If your time ain't come not even a doctor can kill you.

Leigh Stoecker

Death is better than disease.

Henry Wadsworth Longfellow

Those who have the strength and the love to sit with a dying patient in the silence that goes beyond words will know that this moment is neither frightening nor painful, but a peaceful cessation of the functioning of the body.

Elisabeth Kübler-Ross

A long illness seems to be placed between life and death, in order to make death a comfort both to those who die and to those who remain.

Jean de La Bruyère

Many men on the point of an edifying death would be furious if they were suddenly restored to life.

Cesare Pavese

The very word euthanasia is never used because of the madman Hitler . . . . [but] we in Holland know the word means "a mild death, a dignified death." And therefore we use it.

Pieter V. Admiraal

I think very soon the right to die will become the duty to die.

Cecily Saunders

A person is entitled to be buried whole.

Pinchas Stolper, on the use of body parts for transplants and research

I feel as if heaven lay close upon the earth and I between the two, breathing through the eye of a needle.

Amr Ibn Al-As

There is a dignity in dying that doctors should not dare to deny.

Hugh W. Brallier

Death must simply become the discreet but dignified exit of a peaceful person from a helpful society that is not torn, not even overly upset by the idea of a biological transition without significance, without pain or suffering, and ultimately without fear.

Philippe Aries

To die will be an awfully big adventure.

J.M. Barrie

With what shift and pains we come into the world we remember not; but 'tis commonly found no easy matter to get out of it.

Sir Thomas Browne

I am ready to meet my Maker. Whether my Maker is prepared for the ordeal of meeting me is another matter.

Winston Churchill

There is only one ultimate and effectual preventative for the maladies to which flesh is heir, and that is death.

Harvey Cushing

Rather suffer than die is man's motto.

Jean de La Fontaine

If I had the use of my body I would throw it out of the window.

Samuel Beckett

To attempt suicide is a criminal offense. Any man who, of his own will, tries to escape the treadmill to which the rest of us feel chained incites our envy, and therefore our fury. We do not suffer him to go unpunished.

Alexander Chase

Suicide is the worst form of murder, because it leaves no opportunity for repentance.

John Churton Collins

It is against the law to commit suicide in this man's town . . . although what the law can do to a guy who commits suicide I am never able to figure out.

Damon Runyon

I take it that no man is educated who has never dallied with the thoughts of suicide.

William James

I have been half in love with easeful Death.

John Keats

The doctors said at the time that she couldn't live more than a fortnight, and she's been trying ever since to see if she could. Women are so opinionated.

Saki

It is the duty of a doctor to prolong life and it is not his duty to prolong the act of dying.

Horder Thomas

Life was a funny thing that occurred on the way to the grave.

Quentin Crisp

Death is one of the few things that can be done as easily lying down.

Woody Allen

Dying is something ghastly, as being born is something ridiculous.

George Santayana

The body is not a permanent dwelling, but a sort of inn (with a brief sojourn at that) which is to be left behind when one perceives that one is a burden to the host.

Seneca

As a well-spent day brings happy sleep, so life well used brings happy death.

Leonardo da Vinci

There's nothing certain in man's life but this:
That he must lose it.

Edward Bulwer-Lytton

Teach me to live, that I may dread
The grave as little as my bed.

Thomas Ken

The act of dying too is one of the acts of life.

Marcus Aurelius

Ignore death until the last moment; then when it can't be
ignored any longer have yourself squirted full of morphia and
shuffle off in a corner.

Aldous Huxley

Death is the greatest kick of all, that's why they save it for last.

Robert Raisner

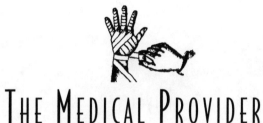

THE MEDICAL PROVIDER

As a young man, the British poet laureate Alfred, Lord Tennyson was afflicted with a painful attack of piles. Accepting advice, he visited a young but well-known proctologist and was so successfully treated that for many years Tennyson had no further trouble.

However, after he had become a famous poet and had been raised to the peerage, he suffered a further attack. Revisiting the proctologist, he expected to be recognized as the former patient who had become the great poet. The proctologist, however, gave no signs of recognition.

It was only when the noble lord had bent over for examination that the proctologist exclaimed, "Ah, Tennyson!"

Physicians

The people in this world put on a tremendous show, and doctors have a front row seat.

Carl Augustus Hamann

Probably to no other are the strengths and weakness of humanity so completely laid bare.

James G. Mumford

A priest sees people at their best, a lawyer at their worst, but a doctor sees them as they really are.

Proverb

Who would become a physician if he could foresee the hardships which are in store for him?

Johann Wolfgang von Goethe

Physicians and public health officials, like soldiers, are always equipped to fight the last war.

René J. Dubos

A man of very moderate ability may be a good physician, if he devotes himself faithfully to the work.

Oliver Wendell Holmes

It is a good idea to "shop around" before you settle on a doctor. Ask about the condition of his Mercedes. Ask about the competence of his mechanic. Don't be shy! After all, you're paying for it.

Dave Barry

How does one become a good doctor? . . . As I understand it a good doctor is one who is shrewd in diagnosis and wise in treatment; but, more than that, he is a person who never spares himself in the interest of his patients; and in addition he is a man who studies the patient not only as a case but also as an individual . . . . The good doctor, whether general practitioner or specialist, is also a man who studies the patient's personality as well as his disease.

Hugh Cairns

Doctors are men who prescribe medicines of which they know little, to cure diseases of which they know less, in human beings of whom they know nothing.

Voltaire

Whenever a doctor cannot do good, he must be kept from doing harm.

Hippocrates

The dedicated physician is constantly striving for a balance between personal, human values, scientific realities and the inevitabilities of God's will.

David Allman

Doctors will have more lives to answer for in the next world than even we generals.

Napoleon Bonaparte

Medical scientists are nice people, but you should not let them treat you.

August Bier

If the clinician, as observer, wishes to see things as they really are, he must make a *tabula rasa* of his mind and proceed without any preconceived notions whatever.

Jean Martin Charcot

The superior doctor prevents sickness;
The mediocre doctor attends to impending sickness;
The inferior doctor treats actual sickness.

Chinese proverb

There is a great difference between a good physician and a bad one; yet very little between a good one and none at all.

Arthur Young

When a doctor does go wrong he is the first of criminals. He has nerve and he has knowledge.

Arthur Conan Doyle

There are only two sorts of doctors: those who practice with their brains, and those who practice with their tongues.

William Osler

Foolish is the doctor who despises the knowledge acquired by the ancients.

Hippocrates

It is not the number of nervous diseases and patients that has grown, but the number of doctors able to study the diseases.

Anton Chekhov

My doctor is nice; every time I see him I'm ashamed of what I think of doctors in general.

Mignon McLaughlin

Doctors overawe us with their power over life and death and their unintelligible handwriting.

David Hapgood

I wonder why ye can always read a doctor's bill an' ye niver can read his purscription.

Finley Peter Dunne

The doctor has been taught to be interested not in health but in disease. What the public is taught is that health is the cure for disease.

Ashley Montagu

A doctor is a person who still has his adenoids, tonsils, and appendix.

Laurence J. Peter

A smart mother makes often a better diagnosis than a poor doctor.

August Bier

Physicians must discover the weaknesses of the human mind, and even condescend to humour them, or they will never be called in to cure the infirmities of the body.

Charles C. Colton

The blunders of a doctor are felt not by himself but by others.

Ar-Rumi

My dear old friend King George V always told me that he would never have died but for that vile doctor.

Margot Asquith

Doctors and undertakers
Fear epidemics of good health.

Gerald Barzan

Temperance and labour are the two real physicians of man: labour sharpens his appetite and temperance prevents his abusing it.

Jean Jacques Rousseau

As long as men are liable to die and are desirous to live, a physician will be made fun of, but he will be well paid.

Jean de La Bruyère

A doctor wastes no time with patients; and if you have to die, he will put the business through quicker than anybody else.

Molière

So many come to the sickroom thinking of themselves as men of science fighting disease and not as healers with a little knowledge helping nature to get a sick man well.

Auckland Geddes

No doctor takes pleasure in the health even of his friends.

Michel de Montaigne

It is very difficult to slow down. The practice of medicine is like the heart muscle's contraction—it's all or none.

Bela Schick

General practice is not for everybody, and especially not for romantic refugees from big city life.

Robert P. Andrews

The true physician does not preach repentance; he offers absolution.

H.L. Mencken

Some patients, though conscious that their condition is perilous, recover their health simply through their contentment with the goodness of the physician.

Hippocrates

I suppose one has a greater sense of intellectual degradation after an interview with a doctor than from any human experience.

Alice James

Doctors should never talk to patients about anything but medicine. When doctors talk politics, economics or sports, they reveal themselves to be ordinary mortals, idiots like the rest of us.

Andy Rooney

Physicians ought not to give their judgment of religion, for the same reason that butchers are not admitted to be jurors upon life and death.

Jonathan Swift

The finger should be kept on the pulse at least until the hundredth beat in order to judge of its kind and character; the friends standing round will be all the more impressed because of the delay, and physician's words will be received with just that much more attention.

Archimathaeus

It is seldom a medical man has true religious views—there is too much pride of intellect.

George Eliot

A physician and a priest ought not to belong to any particular nation, and be divested of all political opinions.

Napoleon Bonaparte

Who ever saw a doctor use the prescription of his colleagues without cutting out or adding something?

Michel de Montaigne

Only the doctor and the dramatist enjoy the rare privilege of charging us for the annoyance they give us.

Santiago Ramon y Cajal

It is unnecessary—perhaps dangerous—in medicine to be too clever.

Robert Hutchinson

A physician who is a lover of wisdom is the equal to a god.

Hippocrates

To prevent disease, to relieve suffering and to heal the sick—this is our work.

William Osler

The common people say that physicians are the best class of people who kill other men in the most polite and courteous manner.

John of Salisbury

The doctors allow one to die, the charlatans kill.

Jean de La Bruyère

English physicians kill you, the French let you die.

William Lamb

This is where the strength of the physician lies, be he a quack, a homeopath, or an allopath. He supplies the perennial demand for comfort, the craving for sympathy that every human sufferer feels.

Leo Tolstoy

A doctor must work eighteen hours a day and seven days a week. If you cannot console yourself to this, get out of the profession.

Martin H. Fischer

"I haven't got time to be sick!" he said. "People need me." For he was a country doctor, and he did not know what it was to spare himself.

Don Marquis

I love doctors and hate their medicine.

Walt Whitman

The face of a physician, like that of a diplomatist, should be impenetrable.

Oliver Wendell Holmes, Sr.

A physician is judged by the three *A*s,
Ability, Availability and Affability.

Paul Reznikoff

He would have been known to the world as a Patriot, had he not been known as something greater—a Physician.

Inscription on a statue of Dr. W.E.B. Davis

That physician will hardly be thought very careful of the health of others who neglects his own.

Galen

The most tragic thing in the world is a sick doctor.

George Bernard Shaw

The physician is an instrument on whom the emotions are played continuously during his waking hours and that is not too good for any man.

Merrill Moore

It is extremely difficult for a physician who puts too much trust in what he reads to form a proper decision from what he sees.

Andrew Boorde

The physician should look upon the patient as a besieged city and try to rescue him with every means that art and science place at his command.

Alexander of Tralles

There is nothing as pleasing to a graying medicine man as the opportunity of slapping a dunce-cap on the young of science.

Ben Hecht

I prefer to have my reward in the gratitude of my patients.

James Young Simpson

A richer pleasure, earth cannot afford
Than when it is your lot, a friend to save
From sinking down to his untimely grave.

Samuel Bartlett Parris

By doing good to humanity with his professional skill, a physician achieves glory, and acquires the plaudits of the good and the wise in this life, and shall live in Paradise in the next.

Sushruta

It is the office of the practitioner to treat safely, speedily, and pleasantly.

Asclepiades

It is as much of the business of a physician to alleviate pain, and to smooth the avenues of death, when unavoidable, as to cure diseases.

John Gregory

The one mark of maturity, especially in a physician, and perhaps it is even rarer in a scientist, is the capacity to deal with uncertainty.

William B. Bean

The doctor is a person who has been trained to think, to observe critically, and to realize that a human being is not a conglomeration of integrated complex systems, but an individual with a personality of his own.

William A.R. Thomson

A true physician is a scientific scholar of human biology who practices his profession as a perceptive humanist.

Dana W. Atchley

Observation, Reason, Human understanding, Courage; these make the physician.

Martin H. Fischer

He who combines the knowledge of physiology and surgery, in addition to the artistic side of his subject, reaches the highest ideal in medicine.

Theodor Billroth

Do not think too much of the dignity of your profession or what it is beneath you to do. It is a moral disorder.

S. Weir Mitchell

The physician himself must be productive, if he really intends to heal; if he is not so, he will only succeed now and then, as if by chance; but, on the whole, he will be only a bungler.

Johann Wolfgang von Goethe

The typical medical man is ignorant of his own simple medicine and puts himself in the hands of unlearned apothecaries.

Roger Bacon

The dignity of a physician requires that he should look healthy, and as plump as nature intended him to be; Then he must be clean in person, well dressed, and anointed with sweet-smelling unguents that are not in any way suspicious.

Hippocrates

The medical profession is not different from any other: its members are, for the most part, ordinary empty-headed dolts, ready to see what is not there and to deny the obvious.

Thomas Mann

My friend, if a doctor did himself what he advises others to do or bade them do the same as he does, he would either suffer in health or in estate.

Roger Bacon

Doctors have a sense for things unseen and complications unstated.

Ben Hecht

On the whole the doctors I have known have been amongst the finest men of my acquaintance . . . . their generosity far surpasses what I have found in any other profession.

William Ralph Inge

Physicians are in general the most amiable companions and the best friends, as well as the most learned men I know.

Alexander Pope

As with eggs, there is no such thing as a poor doctor; doctors are either good or bad.

Fuller Albright

You [doctors] have, and always will be, exposed to the contempt of the gifted amateur—the gentleman who knows by intuition everything that it has taken you years to learn.

Rudyard Kipling

The most conspicuous change in the behavior of the doctor is that nowadays he is usually in such a hurry that he is less accessible and less communicative.

James Howard Means

The talent for secrecy is highly developed among doctors who, even with nothing to conceal, are often as close mouthed as old-fashioned bomb throwers on their way to a rendezvous.

Ben Hecht

Make it compulsory for a doctor using a brass plate to have inscribed on it, in addition to the letters indicating his qualifications, the words "Remember that I too am mortal."

George Bernard Shaw

I have often remarked that, though a physician is sometimes blamed very unjustly, it is quite as common for him to get more credit than he is fairly entitled to; so that he has not, on the whole, any right to complain.

James Jackson

After all, a doctor is just to put your mind at rest.

Petronius

We were lucky in our Medical Heads. Two of them are brutes and four are angels—for this is a work which makes angels or devils of men.

Florence Nightingale

Every physician must be rich in knowledge, and not only of that which is written in books; his patients should be his book, they will never mislead him.

Paracelsus

It is our duty to remember at all times and anew that medicine is not only a science, but also the art of letting our own individuality interact with the individuality of the patient.

Albert Schweitzer

Like a picket at the outposts, the doctor must be ever on call.

Karl Marx

A country doctor needs more brains to do his work passably than the 50 greatest industrialists in the world require.

Walter B. Pitkin

But a doctor who has gone into lonely and discouraged homes, where there was fear for the sick and no one else at hand to administer remedy, and give hope, can really say, "I amount to something. I'm worthwhile."

Carlton K. Matson

All knowledge attains its ethical value and its human significance only by the humane sense in which it is employed. Only a good man can be a great physician.

Hermann Nothnagel

■

Specialists

Specialist: a man who knows more and more about less and less.

William J. Mayo

If the social status of a urologist, a nephrologist, a gastroenterologist, can send a wistful moment through the thoughts of a family practitioner, that is nothing compared with this hovering ghost, this image afloat above the family practitioner's head: Superdoc, the Great American GP, omniscient, ubiquitous.

John McPhee

If there was no such thing as tennis, cardiologists would have had to invent it.

Laurence J. Peter

A medical chest specialist is long-winded about the short-winded.

Kenneth T. Bird

Pediatricians eat because children don't.

Meyer A. Perlstein

If you have more surgeons, you'll get more surgery. If you have more internists, you'll get more lab tests.

John Wennberg

A general practitioner can no more become a specialist than an old shoe can become a dancing slipper. Both have developed habits which are immutable.

Frank Kittredge Paddock

Patients consult so-called authorities. And I have become one also. Yet, we don't know more than the others. We are only the prey of hypochondriacs.

August Bier

To my sons: Whatever specialty they follow, may they never forget to be doctors.

Harry E. Mock

Every specialist, whatever his profession, skill or business may be, can improve his performance by broadening his base.

Wilder Penfield

An expert is a man who tells you a simple thing in a confused way in such a fashion as to make you think the confusion is your own fault.

William B. Castle

There are probably as many "kindly old specialists" as there are "kindly old family physicians."

Robert H. Evert

Popular psychology is a mass of cant, of slush and of superstition worthy of the most flourishing days of the medicine man.

John Dewey

The consultant's first obligation is to the patient, not to his brother physician.

Burton J. Hendrick

It is relatively easy to become a competent specialist, but it is much more difficult to become a good doctor—and it takes much longer.

William Doolin

We anatomists are like the porters in Paris, who are acquainted with the narrowest and most distant streets, but who know nothing of what takes place in the houses.

Bernard Le Bovier de Fontenelle

You will have to learn many tedious things . . . which you will forget the moment you have passed your final examination, but in anatomy it is better to have learned and lost than never to have learned at all.

W. Somerset Maugham

Dermatologists make rash judgments.

Patricia Majewski

A male gynecologist is like an auto mechanic who has never owned a car.

Carrie Snow

Those in the United States who, by and large, have the best medical care and advice readily available to them at the least expense are the families of the specialists in internal medicine. These families use less medicine and undergo less surgery on the whole than any other group, rich or poor.

Edward C. Lambert

I have so little sex appeal that my gynecologist calls me "sir."

Joan Rivers

Pediatricians are men of little patients.

Shelby Friedman

Ugliness is a point of view; an ulcer is wonderful to a pathologist.

Austin O'Malley

Psychiatry

The mind, like a sick body, can be healed and changed by medicine.

Lucretius

The care of the human mind is the most noble branch of medicine.

Aloysius Sieffert

Man's task is to become conscious of the contents that press upward from the unconscious . . . . As far as we can discern, the sole purpose of human existence is to kindle a light in the darkness of mere being.

Carl Jung

If the nineteenth century was the age of the editorial chair, ours is the century of the psychiatrist's couch.

Marshall McLuhan

A psychiatrist has to be a person who commits himself to making a person better. Nothing should be too menial for a psychiatrist to do.

Willibald Nagler

One should only see a psychiatrist out of boredom.

Muriel Spark

The practicing psychotherapist is perhaps better qualified than other serious human beings to discuss boredom.

Victor Altzhul

Psychiatrists are often amusing company, especially when they are drunk.

Al Capp

Men will always be mad and those who think they can cure them are the maddest of all.

Voltaire

Show me a sane man and I will cure him for you.

Carl Jung

Among the millions of nerve cells that clothe parts of the brain there runs a thread. It is the thread of time, the thread that has run through each succeeding wakeful hour of the individual's past life.

Wilder G. Penfield

The relation between psychiatrists and other kinds of lunatic is more or less the relation of a convex folly to a concave one.

Karl Kraus

Anybody who goes to see a psychiatrist ought to have his head examined.

Samuel Goldwyn

Psychoanalysis makes quite simple people feel they're complex.

S.N. Behrman

Psychoanalysis has changed American psychiatry from a diagnostic to a therapeutic science, not because so many patients are cured by the psychoanalytic technique, but because of the new understanding of psychiatric patients it has given us and the new and different concepts of illness and health.

Karl A. Menninger

The repressed memory is like a noisy intruder being thrown out of the concert hall. You can throw him out, but he will bang on the door and continue to disturb the concert. The analyst opens the door and says, "If you promise to behave yourself, you can come back in."

Theodor Reik

The creative person is both more primitive and more cultivated, more destructive, and more constructive, a lot madder and a lot saner, than the average person.

John V. Basmajian

In the office there was an old, soft, and worn blue velvet couch, above which a hundred thousand dissected dreams floated in the peaceful, still air.

Ann Roiphe

A psychiatrist is a person who owns a couch and charges you for lying on it.

Edwin Brock

If we admit our depression openly and freely, those around us get from it an experience of freedom rather than the depression itself.

Rollo May

You handle depression in much the same way you handle a tiger . . . . If depression is creeping up and must be faced, learn something about the nature of the beast: You may escape without a mauling.

R. W. Shepherd

There is no perfect solution to depression, nor should there be. And odd as this may sound . . . we should be glad of that. It keeps us human.

Lesley Hazelton

Psychiatry enables us to correct our faults by confessing our parents' shortcomings.

Laurence J. Peter

Daughters go into analysis hating their fathers, and come out hating their mothers. They never come out hating themselves.

Laurie Jo Wojcik

The old philosophy was that parents, especially mothers, caused their kids to become schizophrenic. Now we see that when a kid is this crazy, he'll make the family begin to seem crazy.

John Talbott

Being a good psychoanalyst, in short, has the same disadvantage as being a good parent: The children desert one as they grow up.

Morton Hunt

We will learn to think of ourselves, our personalities, as an orchestra of chemical voices in our heads.

Arnold J. Mandell

Mental health problems do not affect three or four out of every five persons but one out of one.

William Menninger

Fortunately, analysis is not the only way to resolve inner conflicts. Life itself remains a very effective therapist.

Karen Horney

Psychoanalysis is the disease it purports to cure.
Karl Kraus

Psychoanalysis is a permanent fad.
Peter de Vries

The man who once cursed his fate, now, curses himself—and pays his psychoanalyst.
John W. Gardner

A neurotic is the man who builds a castle in the air. A psychotic is the man who lives in it. And a psychiatrist is the man who collects the rents.
Robert Webb-Johnstone

He is always called a nerve specialist because it sounds better, but everyone knows he's a sort of janitor in a looney bin.

P.G. Wodehouse

Anybody who is 25 or 30 years old has physical scars from all sorts of things, from tuberculosis to polio. It's the same with the mind.

Ralph Kaufman

Analysts keep having to pick away at the scab that the patient tries to form between himself and the analyst to cover over his wounds. The analyst keeps the surface raw, so that the wound will heal properly.

Janet Malcolm

You know what happens to scar tissue. It's the strongest part of your skin.

Michael R. Mantell

Dreaming permits each and every one of us to be quietly and safely insane every night of our lives.

William C. Dement

The inmates are ghosts whose dreams have been murdered.

Jill Johnston, on psychiatric wards

An asylum for the sane would be empty in America.

George Bernard Shaw

I have myself spent nine years in a lunatic asylum and have never suffered from the obsession of wanting to kill myself; but I know that each conversation with a psychiatrist in the morning, made me want to hang myself because I knew I could not strangle him.

Anotonian Artaud

A crowd is a device for indulging ourselves in a kind of temporary insanity by all going crazy together.

Everett Dean Martin

A reservoir of rage exists in each person, waiting to burst out. We fantasize about killing or humiliating our boss or the guy who took our parking space. It is only by growing up in a civilized society of law that we learn the idea of proportionate response.

Ed Magnuson

A psychiatrist is the next man you start talking to after you start talking to yourself.

Fred Allen

Psychiatrist: A man who asks you a lot of expensive questions your wife asks you for nothing.

Sam Bardell

No man is a hero to his wife's psychiatrist.

Eric Berne

Psychoanalysis is spending 40 dollars an hour to squeal on your mother.

Mike Connolly

It is sometimes best to slip over thoughts and not go the bottom of them.

Marie de Sévigné

He was meddling too much in my private life.

Tennessee Williams, on why he stopped seeing his psychoanalyst

I do not have a psychiatrist and I do not want one, for the simple reason that if he listened to me long enough, he might become disturbed.

James Thurber

Psychoanalysts love their insights. They are like gifts they give to themselves.

David S. Viscott

Why should I tolerate a perfect stranger at the bedside of my mind?

Vladimir Nabokov

After twelve years of therapy my psychiatrist said something that brought tears to my eyes. He said, "No hablo inglés."

Ronnie Shakes

Dentistry

Brush them and floss them and take them to the dentist, and they will stay with you. Ignore them, and they'll go away.

American Dental Association

It is necessary to clean the teeth frequently, more especially after meals, but not on any account with a pin, or the point of a penknife, and it must never be done at table.

St. Jean Baptiste de la Salle

If God meant us to eat sugar he wouldn't have invented dentists.

Ralph Nader

Tooth decay was a perennial national problem that meant a mouthful of silver for patients, and for dentists a pocketful of gold.

Claudia Wallis

We all basically go back to being a child when we're in a dentist's chair.

Arthur Benjamin

Every tooth in a man's head is more valuable than a diamond.

Miguel de Cervantes

I'll dispose of my teeth as I see fit, and after they've gone, I'll get along. I started off living on gruel, and by God, I can always go back to it again.

S.J. Perelman

For there was never yet philosopher
That could endure the toothache patiently.

William Shakespeare

The man with toothache thinks everyone happy whose teeth are sound.

George Bernard Shaw

To lose a lover or even a husband or two during the course of one's life can be vexing. But to lose one's teeth is a catastrophe.

Hugh Wheeler

Why is it only teeth that decay . . . . You don't always have to go to the doctor's to have holes in your arms stopped up, do you?

Alan Bennett

That dear little baby tooth, with a small tag attached, reading: "The first bicuspid that little Willie lost. Extracted from Daddy's wrist on April 5, 1887."

W.C. Fields

You can't fully comprehend the phrase "million-dollar smile" until you've had a child in orthodontic braces.

Jean Walter

In my youth, once, when I had a really exquisite toothache, I suddenly realized that my tooth had temporarily become the centre of the universe, that its outcries were more important than anything else, and that I would do absolutely anything to placate it.

Otto Friedrich

A dentist at work in his vocation always looks down in the mouth.

George Prentice

She laughs at everything you say. Why? Because she has fine teeth.

Benjamin Franklin

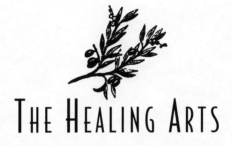

THE HEALING ARTS

The doctor finally reached his table at a dinner, after breaking away from a woman who sought advice on a health problem.

"Do you think I should send her a bill?" the doctor asked a lawyer who sat next to him.

"Why not?" the lawyer replied. "You rendered professional services by giving advice."

"Thanks," the physician said. "I think I'll do that."

When the doctor went to his office the next day to send the bill to the woman, he found a letter from the lawyer. It read: "For legal services, $50."

Ethics

The trouble is not in science but in the uses men make of it. Doctor and layman alike must learn wisdom in their employment of science, whether this applies to atom bombs or blood transfusion.

Wilder Penfield

All who are benefited by community life, especially the physician, owe something to the community.

Charles H. Mayo

The purpose of medicine is to prevent significant disease, to decrease pain, and to postpone death when it is meaningful to do so. Technology has to support these goals—if not, it may even be counterproductive.

Joel J. Nobel

The technology of medicine has outrun its sociology.

Henry E. Sigerist

I fear we are developing a group of competent technicians, treating disease, but not treating the whole patient. All medicine is judgment. I can bring anybody in off the street and teach him how to cut and sew in three months. It is knowing *when* to operate and *when not* to operate that matters.

Alton Ochsner

The twentieth century will be remembered chiefly, not as an age of political conflicts and technical inventions, but as an age in which human society dared to think of the health of the whole human race as a practical objective.

Arnold Toynbee

Euthanasia is a long, smooth-sounding word, and it conceals its danger as long, smooth words do, but the danger is there, nevertheless.

Pearl S. Buck

To save a man's life against his will is the same as killing him.

Horace

Research

Research is the process of going up alleys to see if they're blind.

Marston Bates

Louis Pasteur's theory of germs is a ridiculous fiction. How do you think that these germs in the air can be numerous enough to develop into all these organic infusions? If that were true, they would be numerous enough to form a thick fog, as dense as iron.

Pierre Pochet

Painstaking detective work by medical researchers is producing mounting evidence that environmental impurities in man's habitat are the primary cause of most cancer.

Peter J. Bernstein

You can't make a baby in a month by getting nine women pregnant.

Anonymous

I was on a hunt for 30 years. I wore a laboratory gown, not a Maine guide's red wool jacket.

George D. Snell

Many persons nowadays seem to think that any conclusion must be very scientific if the arguments in favor of it are derived from twitching of frogs' legs—especially if the frogs are decapitated—and that, on the other hand, any doctrine chiefly vouched for by the feelings of human beings—with heads on their shoulders—must be benighted and superstitious.

William James

A drug is a substance that when injected into a guinea pig produces a scientific paper.

Anonymous

It is now proved beyond doubt that smoking is one of the leading causes of statistics.

Fletcher Knebel

Did you hear what the white rat said to the other white rat? "I've got that psychologist so well trained that every time I ring the bell he brings me something to eat."

David Mercer

We're all of us guinea pigs in the laboratory of God. Humanity is just a work in progress.

Tennessee Williams

Some of the papers presented at today's medical meeting tell us what we already know, but in a much more complicated manner.

Alphonse Raymond Dochez

Not the possession of truth but the effort in struggling to attain it brings joy to the researcher.

Gotthold Lessing

The observer listens to Nature; the experimenter questions and forces her to unveil herself.

Georges Cuvier

Research, though toilsome, is easy; imaginative vision, though delightful, is difficult.

A.C. Bradley

You do one experiment in medicine to convince yourself, then 99 more to convince others.

Alphonse Raymond Dochez

No warm, sympathetic person is frozen by research experience, nor is a cold tactless individual thawed by general practice.

Dana W. Atchley

The faculties developed by doing research are those most needed in diagnosis.

Francis Heed Adler

A man may do research for the fun of doing it but he cannot expect to be supported for the fun of doing it.

J. Howard Brown

He uses statistics as a drunken man uses lampposts—for support rather than for illumination.

Andrew Lang

Every sensible person promptly associates the term "statistics" with the thought: "This is a bunch of lies."

August Bier

Statistics . . . will prove anything, even the truth.

Berkeley Moynihan

To discover and teach are distinct functions; they are also distinct gifts, and are not commonly found united in the same person.

John Henry Newman

A man who has a theory which he tries to fit to facts is like a drunkard who tries his key haphazard in door after door, hoping to find one it fits.

J. Chalmers Da Costa

In many laboratories reprints are displayed much as if they were campaign medals on show in a general's drawing room.

John Maddox

One of the things the average doctor doesn't have time to do is catch up with the things he didn't learn in school, and one of the things he didn't learn in school is the nature of human society, its purpose, its history, and its needs . . . . If medicine is necessarily a mystery to the average man, nearly everything else is necessarily a mystery to the average doctor.

Milton Mayer

Every great advance in science has issued from a new audacity of imagination.

John Dewey

The first qualification for a physician is hopefulness.

James Little

If there weren't so many professors, medicine would be much easier.

August Bier

One goes through school, college, medical school, and one's internship learning little or nothing about goodness but a good deal about success.

Ashley Montagu

Other books have been written by men physicians . . . one would suppose in reading them that women possess but one class of physical organs, and that these are always diseased. Such teaching is pestiferous, and tends to cause and perpetuate the very evils it professes to remedy.

Mary Ashton Livermore

The student is to collect and evaluate facts. The facts are locked up in the patient.

Abraham Flexner

Medicine is the one place where all the show is stripped of the human drama. You, as doctors, will be in a position to see the human race stark naked—not only physically, but mentally and morally as well.

Martin H. Fischer

The education of the doctor which goes on after he has his degree is, after all, the most important part of his education.

John Shaw Billings

Medical education is not completed at the medical school: it is only begun.

William H. Welch

One thing seems certain—if we taught and examined less, our students would learn more. If we add anything further to the medical curriculum let it be spare time.

C.C. Okell

I respect faith but doubt is what gets you an education.

Wilson Mizner

Official academies are more likely to exhibit enthusiasm over the improvements of the commonplace than to recognize the unexpected when it is first brought to them.

René J. Dubos

In teaching the medical student the primary requisite is to keep him awake.

Chevalier Jackson

If you want to get out of medicine the fullest enjoyment, be students all your lives.

David Riesman

Medical instruction does not exist to provide individuals with an opportunity of learning how to make a living, but in order to make possible the protection of the health of the public.

Rudolf Virchow

The pleasure of a physician is little, the gratitude of patients is rare . . . but these things will never deter the student who feels the call within him.

Theodor Billroth

Keep always bright by using the desire to serve that all of you expressed when you sought admission to the study of medicine.

Kenneth M. Lynch

The paths of pain are thine. Go forth with healing and with hope.

John Greenleaf Whittier

The Patient

One of the essential qualities of the clinician is interest in humanity, for the secret of the care of the patient is in caring for the patient.

Francis Weld Peabody

It is the human touch after all that counts for most in our relation with our patients.

Robert Tuttle Morris

The physician must generalize the disease, and individualize the patient.

Christoph Wilhelm Hufeland

The human body is a machine which winds its own springs; the living image of perpetual movement.

Julien Offroy de la Mettrie

Every stress leaves an indelible scar, and the organism pays for its survival after a stressful situation by becoming a little older.

Hans Selye

The human body . . . indeed is like a ship; its bones being the stiff standing-rigging, and the sinews the small running ropes, that manage all the motions.

Herman Melville

The patient is not likely to recover who makes the doctor his heir.

Thomas Fuller

Don't touch the patient—state first what you see.

William Osler

There's another advantage of being poor—a doctor will cure you faster.

Frank McKinney Hubbard

Let no one suppose that the words "doctor" and "patient" can disguise from the parties the fact that they are employer and employee.

George Bernard Shaw

After two days in the hospital, I took a turn for the nurse.

W.C. Fields

Doctors think a lot of patients are cured who have simply quit in disgust.

Don Herold

While the patient wants the best and most modern treatment available, he is also badly in need of the old-fashioned friend that a doctor has always personified and which you must continue to be.

Gunnar Gundersen

Remember to cure the patient as well as the disease.

Alvan Barach

The patient is always the ultimate source of knowledge.

Philip Bonnet

Patients with migraines know precisely when and how often and how long their headaches strike. They often come in with long lists. When you have a patient with lists, you have a patient with migraine.

Seymour Diamond

What is most interesting in family practice is not what the problem is but what motivates people to seek help for it. Something in the family, a hidden factor, will make the mundane interesting.

Sandy Burstein

There is only one cardinal rule: One must always listen to the patient.

Oliver Sacks

The doctor may also learn more about the illness from the way the patient tells the story than from the story itself.

James B. Herrick

Ordinarily he is insane, but he has lucid moments when he is only stupid.

Heinrich Heine

It is not a case we are treating; it is a living, palpitating, alas, too often suffering fellow creature.

John Brown

The Best Medicine

A patient complaining of melancholy consulted with the British physician John Abernethy.

After an examination Abernethy pronounced, "You need amusement. Go and hear the comedian Grimaldi; he will make you laugh and that will be better for you than any drugs."

Said the patient, "I am Grimaldi."

First, the patient, second the patient, third the patient, fourth the patient, fifth the patient, and then maybe comes science. We first do everything for the patient; science can wait, research can wait.

Béla Schick

Never believe what a patient tells you his doctor has said.

William Jenner

Before you tell the "truth" to the patient, be sure you know the "truth," and that the patient wants to hear it.

Richard Clarke Cabot

I haven't asked you to make me young again. All I want is to go on getting older.

Konrad Adenauer

Once someone has chosen to fall ill, he has to apply for the role of patient; he auditions for the part by reciting his complaints as vividly and convincingly as he can.

Jonathan Miller

The treatment of a disease may be entirely impersonal; the care of a patient must be completely personal.

Francis Weld Peabody

We now feel we can cure the patient without his fully understanding what made him sick. We are no longer so interested in peeling the onion as in changing it.

Franz Alexander

One must not count upon all of his patients being willing to steal in order to pay doctor's bills.

Robert Tuttle Morris

Let your entrance into the sick room decrease, not increase, the irritability of your patient.

Martin H. Fisher

Nothing is too good for the patient, provided it doesn't involve any extra effort on my part.

Thomas Huxley

Don't refer a patient to a psychiatrist as if you are telling him to go to hell.

Walter Lincoln Palmer

The patient's family will never forgive a guarantee of cure that failed and the patient will not let the physician forget a pronouncement of incurability if he is so fortunate as to survive.

George T. Pack

The patient may well be safer with a physician who is naturally wise than with one who is artificially learned.

Sir Theodore Fox

There are only two classes of mankind in the world—doctors and patients.

Rudyard Kipling

The patient who consults a great many physicians is likely to have a very confused state of mind.

Rhazes

When I was young, patients were afraid of me; now that I am old, I am afraid of patients.

Johann Peter Frank

The patient should be managed the way the doctor or a member of his family would wish to be treated if he were that patient in that bed at that time.

Robert F. Loeb

It is better to shoot the patient than to shoot the works.

Hugh Cabot

Hospitals

The two places one should always go first class are in hospitals and on ships.

Barbara A. Huff

The very first requirement in a hospital is that it should do the sick no harm.

Florence Nightingale

A hospital should also have a recovery room adjoining the cashier's office.

Francis O'Walsh

Blue Cross Hiltons.
Edgar Berman

One of the most difficult things to contend with in a hospital is the assumption on the part of the staff that because you have lost your gall bladder you have also lost your mind.
Jean Kerr

The ultimate indignity is to be given a bedpan by a stranger who calls you by your first name.
Maggie Kuhn

If you want to be on the staff of a hospital, lad, pretend you're a fool till you're on it.
Lloyd Roberts

Private patients, if they do not like me, can go elsewhere; but the poor devils in the hospital I am bound to take care of.

John Abernethy

That should assure us of at least 45 minutes of undisturbed privacy.

Dorothy Parker, upon pressing her bedside nurse's bell

Regulations of the Philadelphia General Hospital, 1790

Patients may not swear, curse, get drunk, behave rudely or indecently on pain of expulsion after the first admonition. There shall be no card playing or dicing and such patients as are able shall assist in nursing others, washing and ironing linen and cleaning the rooms and such other services as the matron may require.

Medicine is an advancing science and the best hospitals in the world are not those which merely use new knowledge, but those which create it.

Sir George W. Pickering

The purpose of a teaching hospital is to advance knowledge, to train doctors, and to set an example of practice.

Nathaniel Faxon

Hospitals are the temples of medicine. What may not always be possible in private practice must be possible in a hospital. Accidents and delays which might be forgiven in private practice are inexcusable in the hospital.

Henry E. Sigerist

So it was all modern and scientific and well-arranged. You could die very nearly as privately in a modern hospital as you could in the Grand Central Station, and with much better care.

Stephen Vincent Benét

Here, at whatever hour you come, you will find light and help and human kindness.

Inscription on the lamp outside Albert Schweitzer's jungle hospital at Lambarene

First need in the reform of hospitals management? That's easy! The death of all dietitians, and the resurrection of a French chef.

Martin H. Fisher

Life is a hospital in which every patient is possessed by the desire to change his bed.

Charles Baudelaire

The only places where American medicine can fully live up to its possibilities are the teaching hospitals.

Bernard De Voto

Every hospital should have a plaque in the physicians' and students' entrances: "There are some patients whom we cannot help, there are none whom we cannot harm."

Arthur L. Bloomfield

■

SURGERY

A good surgeon operates with his hand, not with his heart.

Alexandre Dumas _pere_

Surgery is the ready motion of steady and experienced hands.

Galen

The first attribute of a surgeon is an insatiable curiosity.

Russell John Howard

In surgery eyes first and most; fingers next and little; tongue last and least.

George Murray Humphry

A possible apprehension now is that the surgeon be sometimes tempted to supplant instead of aiding Nature.

Henry Maudsley

Speed in operating should be the achievement, not the aim, of every surgeon.

Russell John Howard

The feasibility of an operation is not the best indication for its performance.

Henry, Lord Cohen of Birkenhead

Surgery does the ideal thing—it separates the patient from his disease. It puts the patient back to bed and the disease in a bottle.

Logan Clendening

I got the bill for my surgery. Now I know what those doctors were wearing masks for.

James H. Boren

When they operated, I told them to put in a Koufax fastball. They did—but it was a Mrs. Koufax fastball.

Tommy John

When I take up assassination, I shall start with the surgeons in this city and work *up* to the gutter.

Dylan Thomas

In a good surgeon, a hawk's eye; a lion's heart; and a lady's hand.

Leonard Wright

The epithet *beautiful* is used by surgeons to describe an operation which their patients describe as ghastly.

George Bernard Shaw

She got her good looks from her father—he's a plastic surgeon.

Groucho Marx

Anybody who is anybody seems to be getting a lift—by plastic surgery—these days. It's the new world-wide craze that combines the satisfactions of psychoanalysis, massage, and a trip to the beauty salon.

Eugenia Sheppard

Is not plastic surgery an art and the plastic surgeon an artist? The plastic surgeon works with living flesh as his clay, and his work of art is the attempted achievement of normalcy in appearance and function.

Jerome Pierce Webster

The surgeon can cut out the ulcer, but he can't cut out the tensions.

Curtis Vouwie

I have made many mistakes myself; in learning the anatomy of the eye I dare say, I have spoiled a hatful; the best surgeon, like the best general, is he who makes the fewest mistakes.

Astley Paston Cooper

Every surgeon carries about him a little cemetery, in which from time to time he goes to pray, a cemetery of bitterness and regret, of which he seeks the reason for certain of his failures.

Rene Leriche

Pray before surgery, but remember God will not alter a faulty incision.

Arthur H. Keeney

Surgery is always second best. If you can do something else, it's better.

John Kirklin

He who wishes to be a surgeon should go to war.

Hippocrates

The surgeon who is his own physician, though he often has a fool for a colleague, has the happiness of working in an atmosphere of mutual confidence and admiration.

Heneage Ogilvie

Th' incurable cut off, the rest reforme.

Ben Jonson

I would like to see the day when somebody would be appoint-
ed surgeon somewhere who had no hands, for the operative
part is the least part of the work.

Harvey Cushing

There cannot always be fresh fields of conquest by the knife;
there must be portions of the human frame that will ever
remain sacred from its intrusions, at least in the surgeon's
hands. That we have already, if not quite, reached these final
limits, there can be little question. The abdomen, the chest,
and the brain will be forever shut from the intrusion of the wise
and humane surgeon.

John Eric Erichsen

The abolishment of pain in surgery is a chimera. It is absurd to go on seeking it . . . . Knife and pain are two words in surgery that must forever be associated in the consciousness of the patient. To this compulsory combination we shall have to adjust ourselves.

Alfred Velpeau

What Gall!

Supreme Court Justice William J. Brennan felt faint while working at his desk and was rushed to a nearby hospital, where he was diagnosed with pneumonia.

Brennan was then admitted to the hospital where he was found to be suffering from a gall bladder condition as well. Doctors removed it.

Soon thereafter, former Chief Justice Burger was admitted to another hospital with pneumonia. Brennan called him, advising, "Warren, you'd better get out of there quickly. If they think you have pneumonia, they'll take your gall bladder out."

Surgery is the red flower that blooms among the leaves and thorns that are the rest of medicine.

Richard Selzer

■

Treatment

The cure for anything is salt water—sweat, tears, or the sea.

Isak Dinesen

Most things get better by themselves. Most things, in fact, are better by morning.

Lewis Thomas

It is part of the cure to wish to be cured.

Seneca

The more serious the illness, the more important it is for you to fight back, mobilizing all your resources—spiritual, emotional, intellectual, physical.

Norman Cousins

There are no such things as incurable, there are only things for which man has not found a cure.

Bernard Baruch

Diseases come of their own accord,
But *cures* come difficult and hard.

Samuel Butler

A physician is obligated to consider more than a diseased organ, more even than the whole man—he must view the man in his world.

Harvey Cushing

The art of healing comes from nature, not from the physician. Therefore the physician must start from nature, with an open mind.

Paracelsus

There's a greater law than the FDA, and that is an obligation of a doctor to try to do anything he can to save a life when he thinks that there's a chance.

Cecil Vaughn

When you are exhausted from trying to beat the odds against recovery, when you want only to cash in your chips and let them fall where they may, you do not ask your doctor to gamble with your life, but to stop gambling.

Steven Radlauer

It is more important to cure people than to make diagnoses.

August Bier

To learn how to treat disease, one must learn how to recognize it. The diagnosis is the best trump in the scheme of treatment.

Jean Martin Charcot

It is too bad that we cannot cut the patient in half in order to compare two regimens of treatment.

Béla Schick

We don't consider a patient cured when his sprain has healed or he's been restored to a minimal level of functioning. The patient is cured when he can again do the things he loves to do.

Stanley A. Herring

We are too much accustomed to attribute to a single cause that which is the product of several, and the majority of our controversies come from that.

Justus von Liebig

LSD is, if you like, a psychiatric x-ray. With LSD you have no greater vision of the universe than you did before. It no more expands your consciousness than an X-ray expands your lungs when you see them on the screen. All you do is get a better look.

Marvin Ziporyn

We recommend that he take a basic CPR course, but it's hard to argue with success.

Keith Luri, on a man who used a toilet plunger on his father's chest to save his life during a heart attack

A good laugh and a long sleep are the best cures in the doctor's book.

Irish proverb

If you want to clear your system out, sit on a piece of cheese and swallow a mouse.

Johnny Carson

Every businessman over fifty should have a daily nap and nip—a short nap after lunch and a relaxing highball before dinner.

Sara Murray Jordan

Is getting well ever an art
Or art a way to get well?

Robert Lowell

We do not know what we mean by cure because there is a great difference between cure and long-term survival.

Arthur Holleb

Then comes the question, how do drugs, hygiene, and animal magnetism heal? It may be affirmed that they do not heal, but only relieve suffering temporarily, exchanging one disease for another.

Mary Baker Eddy

Saying "Gesundheit" doesn't really help the common cold—
but it's about as good as anything the doctors have come up
with.

Earl Wilson

Whiskey is the most popular of all the remedies that won't cure
a cold.

Jerry Vale

After 30 years' practice, I am fully convinced that two-thirds of
all my patients would have recovered without the use of
physic, or the attendance of a physician.

Christoph Wilhelm Hufeland

Surely every medicine is an innovation, and he that will not
apply new remedies, must expect new evils.

Francis Bacon

The physician's best remedy is *Tincture of Time!*

Bela Schick

The only cure for seasickness is to sit on the shady side of an old brick church in the country.

English sailors' proverb

Speak roughly to your little boy,
      And beat him when he sneezes:
He only does it to annoy.
      Because he knows it teases.

Lewis Carroll

Well, now, there's a remedy for everything except death.

Miguel de Cervantes

When a lot of remedies are suggested for a disease, that means it can't be cured.

Anton Chekhov

Difficult as it may be to cure, it is always easy to poison and to kill.

Elisha Bartlett

I would like to remind those responsible for the treatment of tuberculosis that Keats wrote his best poems while dying of this disease. In my opinion he would never have done so under the influence of modern chemotherapy.

Arthur M. Walker

Keep up the spirits of your patient with the music of the viol and the psaltery, or by forging letters telling of the death of his enemies or (if he be a cleric) by informing him that he has been made a bishop.

Henri de Mondeville

Work is the grand cure of all the maladies and miseries that ever beset mankind.

Thomas Carlyle

She had always found occupation to be one of the best medicines for an afflicted mind.

Eliza Leslie

Visitors' footfalls are like medicine; they heal the sick.

Bantu proverb

It often happens that the sicker man is the nurse to the sounder.

Henry David Thoreau

If you are too fond of new remedies, first you will not cure your patients; secondly, you will have no patients to cure.

Astley Paston Cooper

Because the newer methods of treatment are good, it does not follow that the old ones were bad: for if our honorable and worshipful ancestors had not recovered from their ailments, you and I would not be here today.

Confucius

New medicines, and new methods of cure, always work miracles for a while.

John Armstrong

My sore-throats, you know, are always worse than anybody's.

Jane Austen

I have a perfect cure for a sore throat: cut it.

Alfred Hitchcock

Better a tried remedy than a new-fangled one.

Ambroise Pare

Take a dose of medicine once, and in all probability you will be obliged to take an additional hundred afterwards.

Napoleon Bonaparte

We shall have to learn to refrain from doing things merely because we know how to do them.

Theodore Fox

In treating a patient, let your first thought be to strengthen his natural vitality.

Rhazes

I dressed him and God healed him.

Ambroise Pare

None can speak of a wound with skill, if he hath not a wound felt.

Philip Sidney

Despair is better treated with hope, not dope.

Richard Asher

The desire to take medicine is perhaps the greatest feature
which distinguishes man from animals.

William Osler

The worse about medicine is that one kind makes another necessary.

Elbert Hubbard

The pen is mightier than the sword! The case for prescriptions
rather than surgery.

Marvin Kitman

Modern medicine has made drugs highly legitimate, something
to be taken casually and not only during moments of acute and
certified stress.

William Simon

The pharmaceutical industry is redefining and relabeling as medicinal problems calling for drug intervention a wide range of human behaviors which, in the past, have been viewed as falling within the bounds of the normal trials and tribulations of human existence.

Henry L. Lennard

That great American tabernacle, the medicine cabinet.

Peter Fasolino

Vaccination is the medical sacrament corresponding to baptism.

Samuel Butler

Tranquilizers do not change our environment, nor do they change our personalities. They merely reduce our responsiveness to stimuli . . . once the response has been dulled, the irritating surface noise of living muted or eliminated, the spark and brilliance are also gone.

Indra Devi

What is dangerous about tranquilizers is that whatever peace of mind they bring is packaged peace of mind. Where you buy a pill and buy peace with it, you get conditioned to cheap solutions instead of deep ones.

Max Lerner

This society seems to have swallowed the notion that there is a chemical solution for all problems, including the problem of how to spend one's spare time.

Joel Fort

A man who cannot work without his hypodermic needle is a poor doctor. The amount of narcotic you use is inversely proportional to your skill.

Martin H. Fischer

A miracle drug is any drug that will do what the label says it will do.

Eric Hodgins

The patient, treated on the fashionable theory, sometimes gets well in spite of the medicine. The medicine therefore restored him, and the young doctor receives new courage to proceed in his bold experiments on the lives of his fellow creatures.

Thomas Jefferson

There are no really "safe" biologically active drugs. There are only "safe" physicians.

Harold A. Kaminetzky

Drugs, cataplasms, and whiskey are stupid substitutes for the dignity and potency of divine Mind, and its efficacy to heal.

Mary Baker Eddy

Poisons and medicine are oftentimes the same substance given with different intents.

Peter Mere Latham

It requires a great deal of faith for a man to be cured by his own placebos.

John L. McClenahan

Dr. Simpson's first patient, a doctor's wife in 1847, had been so carried away with enthusiasm that she christened her child, a girl, "Anaesthesia."

Elizabeth Longford

Dr. Snow gave that blessed chloroform and the effect was soothing, quieting, and delightful beyond measure.

Victoria, Queen of England

Orthodox medicine has not found an answer to your complaint. However, luckily for you, I happen to be a quack.

Charles Richter cartoon caption

By quack I mean imposter not in opposition to but in common with physicians.

Horace Walpole

It is better to have recourse to a quack, if he can cure our disorder, although he cannot explain it, than to a physician, if he can explain our disease, but cannot cure it.

Charles C. Colton

To preserve a man alive in the midst of so many chances and hostilities, is as great a miracle as to create him.

Jeremy Taylor

Three natural anaesthetics . . . sleep, fainting, death.

Oliver Wendell Holmes, Sr.

■

Profit and Loss

God heals and the Doctor takes the Fees.

Benjamin Franklin

The threat of a neglected cold is for doctors what the threat of purgatory is for priests—a gold mine.

Nicholas Chamfort

Financial ruin from medical bills is almost exclusively an American disease.

Roul Turley

The very success of medicine in a material way may now threaten the soul of medicine.

Walter Martin

Money-giving is a very good criterion . . . of a person's mental health. Generous people are rarely mentally ill people.

Karl A. Menninger

There are more doctors in a single North Shore medical building than in one entire West Side ghetto.

Jack Starr

Health care is being converted from a social service to an economic commodity, sold in the marketplace and distributed on the basis of who can afford to pay for it.

Arnold Relman

My doctor is wonderful. Once, in 1955, when I couldn't afford an operation, he touched up the x-rays.

Joey Bishop

So we open the kid up, and what do you think we find? Three buttons, a thumb tack, and twenty-seven cents in change . . . . The parents couldn't afford to pay for the operation, so I kept the twenty-seven cents.

Billy Wilder

Our doctor would never really operate unless it was necessary. He was just that way. If he didn't need the money, he wouldn't lay a hand on you.

Herb Shriner

Get your money when the patient is in pain.

Proverb

The doctor demands his fees whether he has killed the illness or the patient.

Polish proverb

A fashionable surgeon, like a pelican, can be recognized by the size of his bill.

J. Chalmers Da Costa

There are two kinds of appendicitis—acute appendicitis and appendicitis for revenue only.

Richard Clarke Cabot

A physician who heals for nothing is worth nothing.

The Talmud

I feel that the greatest reward for doing is the opportunity to do more.

Jonas Salk

When a doctor looks me square in the face and kant see no money in me, than i am happy.

Josh Billings

Most medical men are amateurs at finance, and what is learned comes through bitter experience.

D. Ralph Millard, Jr.

Is there no hope? the sick man said.
The silent doctor shook his head,
And took his leave, with signs of sorrow,
Despairing of his fee tomorrow.

John Gay

A doctor shouldn't have to worry about money! That's one disease he's not trained to fight. It either corrupts him . . . or it destroys him.

Sidney Kingsley

Boys, don't study medicine. By the time you earn your bread, you will have no teeth left to eat it with.

Henry McMurtrie

The medical profession is the only one which a man may enter at any age with some chance of making a living.

W. Somerset Maugham

It is because we have begun to act like merchants, and in many instances to observe the same hours, that the public expects us to be regulated by the same restraints.

John L. McClenahan

■

Lawyers

There was a time when an apple a day kept the doctor away,
but now it's malpractice insurance.

Laurence J. Peter

The animals are not as stupid as one thinks—they
have neither doctors nor lawyers.

L. Docquier

Doctors and lawyers must go to school for
years and years, often with little sleep and
with great sacrifice to their first wives.

Roy Blount, Jr.

The more things doctors are able to do, the more likely that at least a few doctors won't do them. And the result will be more people suing for negligence.

George J. Annas

They learn that once they enter the court, they are in someone else's operating room.

Donald J. Ciaglia, on teaching legal procedures to medical students

Doctors are just the same as lawyers; the only difference is that lawyers merely rob you, whereas doctors rob you and kill you, too.

Anton Chekhov

THE PRACTICE OF MEDICINE

Medicine, the only profession that labours incessantly to destroy the reason for its existence.

James Bryce

There is no greater reward in our profession than the knowledge that God has entrusted us with the physical care of his people.

Elmer Hess

I am interested in physical medicine because my father was. I am interested in medical research because I believe in it. I am interested in arthritis because I have it.

Bernard Baruch

We have not lost faith, but we have transferred it from God to the medical profession.

George Bernard Shaw

Medicine is not a lucrative profession. It is a divine one.

John Coakley Lettsom

Medicine is an occupation for slaves.

Benjamin Rush

Medicine is a noble profession but a damn bad business.

Humphrey Rolleston

If you would die fagged to death like a crow with the king birds after him—be a school-master; if you would wax thin and savage, like a half-fed spider—be a lawyer; if you would go off like an opium-eater in love with your starving delusions—be a doctor.

Oliver Wendell Holmes, Sr.

Benjamin Franklin Advises

To lengthen thy Life, lessen thy Meals.

It is ill Jesting with the Joiner's Tools;
worse with the Doctor's.

Beware of the young doctor and the old barber.

He's the best physician that knows
the worthlessness of the most medicines.

Nothing is more fatal to *Health*, than an *over Care* of it.

There are more old drunkards than old doctors.

The American Medical Association, operating from a platform of negative vigilance, presents no solutions but busily fights each change and then loudly supports it against the next proposal.

John H. Knowles

It takes fifty years from the discovery of a principle in medicine to its adoption in practice.

Martin H. Fischer

I always have to laugh when the AMA claims that doctors have no special powers over people. How many people can tell you to take off your clothes and you'll do it?

Robert S. Mendelsohn

The history of medicine is a story of amazing foolishness and amazing intelligence.

Jerome Tarshis

Good advice is no better than bad advice unless it is taken at the right time.

Danish proverb

Never go to a doctor whose office plants have died.

Erma Bombeck

Medicine may be defined as the art or the science of keeping a patient quiet with frivolous reasons for his illness and amusing him with remedies good or bad until nature kills him or cures him.

Gilles Menage

The best practitioners give to their patients the least medicine.

Frederick Saunders

Nobody in the United States is more than one handshake away from virtually any drug they want to get.

Norman Zinberg

The whole imposing edifice of modern medicine, for all its breathtaking successes, is, like the celebrated Tower of Pisa, slightly off balance. It is frightening how dependent on drugs we are all becoming and how easy it is for doctors to prescribe them as the universal panacea for our ills.

Prince Charles

I will lift up mine eyes unto the pills. Almost everyone takes them, from the humble aspirin to the multi-coloured, king-sized three deckers, which put you to sleep, wake you up, stimulate and soothe you all in one. It is an age of pills.

Malcolm Muggeridge

Grief is itself a medicine.

William Cowper

Medicine is like a woman who changes with the fashions.

August Bier

The aim of medicine is surely not to make men virtuous; it is to safeguard and rescue them from the consequences of their vices.

H.L. Mencken

First farming, next trade, last service, or at least begging; if you cannot obtain alms, learn to be a doctor.

Indian (Marathi) proverb

The joy of medicine is the challenge of making a solid diagnosis, the delight in besting (if only momentarily) an intern or resident, the satisfaction (if rare) of actually helping someone, the sheer cantankerousness of being able to tell the bureaucracy to "stuff it."

Michael J. Halberstam

The place of medicine is in the stream of life, not on its banks.

René Sand

Always give the patient hope, even when death seems at hand.

Ambroise Paré

There is no more contradiction between the science of medicine and the art of medicine than between the science of aeronautics and the art of flying.

Francis Weld Peabody

The medical profession is a noble and pleasant one, though laborious and often full of anxiety.

Andrew James Symington

The prime goal is to alleviate suffering, and not to prolong life. And if your treatment does not alleviate suffering, but only prolongs life, that treatment should be stopped.

Christiaan Barnard

Medicine heals doubts as well as diseases.

Karl Marx

A man need not have grown old in the practice of medicine to bear witness to its having undergone considerable changes.

Peter Mere Latham

Medicine should be practiced as a form of friendship.

Léon Bernard

Medicine: When in good health, make fun of it.

Gustave Flaubert

Index

Alexander, Franz (1891–1964), American physician and psycho-analyst, 214

Allen, Fred (1894–1956), American humorist, 182

Allen, Woody, b. 1935, American comedian and film maker, 43, 54, 135

Allman, David, American Medical Association president, 77, 143

Altzhul, Victor, American psychiatry professor, 173

Amiel, Henri (1821–1881), Swiss poet and philosopher, 73

Amis, Kingsley, b. 1922, British writer, 98

Anderson, J., b. 1926, 71

Andrews, Robert P., b. 1935, 149

Annas, George J., American professor of health law, 256

Archimathaeus, c. 1100, 151

Aries, Philippe, 20th-century writer, 132

Aristotle (384–322 B.C.), Greek philosopher, 51

Armstrong, John (1709–1779), Scottish physician and poet, 34, 241

Armstrong, Neil, b. 1930, American astronaut, 101

Ar-Rumi (1207–1273), Persian poet, 147

Artaud, Antonin (1896–1948), French dramatist, actor, and poet, 181

Asclepiades (3rd century B.C.), Greek poet, 157

Asher, Richard, b. 1912, writer, 243

Askey, Vincent, American Medical Association president, 66, 121

Asquith, Margot (1865–1945), English political figure, 147

Atchley, Dana W., b. 1892, medical writer, 158, 199

Auber, Esprit (1782–1871), French composer, 81

Augustine, St. (354–430), Latin philosopher and religious leader, 67, 118

Aurelius, Marcus (121–180 A.D.), Roman emperor, 137

Austen, Jane (1775–1817), English writer, 241

Bacon, Francis (1561–1626), English philosopher and statesman, 40, 67, 85, 237

Bacon, Roger (1220–1292), English philosopher and scientist, 38, 159, 160

Baden, Michael M., 20th-century medical examiner, 113

Baden-Powell, Robert (1857–1941), English soldier and founder of Boy Scouts, 43

Balzac, Honoré de (1799–1850), French novelist, 47, 86

Barach, Alvan, 20th-century inventor, 86, 88, 210

Bardell, Sam, b. 1915, 182

ABOUT THE AUTHOR

Jess M. Brallier is the son of a dentist and a nurse, and the brother of a physician. He is the author of *The Pessimist's Journal of Very, Very Bad Days, The Really, Really Classy Donald Trump Quiz Book,* and the bestselling *Lawyers and Other Reptiles*. He lives near Boston.